Health Behavior Change

Dedications

SR: To my dear boys, Jacob and Stefan, and my wife Sheila: thank you
PM: To Hugh, with love and thanks
CCB: To Judith, Caitlin and Eva

Commissioning Editor: Alex Mathieson
Project Development Editor: Valerie Dearing
Project Manager: Ewan Halley
Design Direction: Judith Wright

Health Behavior Change
A Guide for Practitioners

Stephen Rollnick BSocSci(Hons) MSc DipClinPsych PhD
Clinical Psychologist and Senior Lecturer, Department of General Practice,
University of Wales, College of Medicine, Cardiff, UK

Pip Mason RGN BSc(Econ) MSocSc
Nurse and Training Consultant, Aquarius, Birmingham, UK

Christopher Butler BA MBChB DCH MRCGP
General Practitioner and Lecturer, Department of General Practice,
University of Wales, College of Medicine, Cardiff, UK

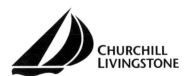

CHURCHILL
LIVINGSTONE

EDINBURGH LONDON NEW YORK PHILADELPHIA SYDNEY TORONTO 1999

CHURCHILL LIVINGSTONE
An imprint of Harcourt Publishers Limited

First published 1999
  Reprinted 2000 (twice)

ISBN 0443 058504

British Library of Cataloguing in Publication Data
A catalogue record for this book is available from the British Library

Library of Congress Cataloging in Publication Data
A catalog record for this book is available from the Library of Congress

Note
Medical knowledge is constantly changing. As new information becomes
available, changes in treatment, procedures, equipment and the use of
drugs become necessary. The editors/authors/contributors and the
publishers have, as far as it is possible, taken care to ensure that the
information given in this text is accurate and up to date. However, readers
are strongly advised to confirm that the information, especially with
regard to drug usage, complies with current legislation and standards of
practice.

The
publisher's
policy is to use
**paper manufactured
from sustainable forests**

Printed in China

Contents

PREFACE

Conventional wisdom can oversimplify the relationship between practitioners and their patients. It is assumed that patients report a set of symptoms, and that practitioners diagnose and treat. However, many encounters in health practice are not so simple, none more so than those in which symptoms or the threat of them are related to the lifestyle or behavior of the patient. Practitioners are then faced with the need to reveal this to the patient and to suggest changes, often radical, to their lifestyles. This is what we mean by a consultation about health behavior change and which is the subject of this book.

This book is written primarily for healthcare professionals (e.g. nurses, doctors, midwives, physical therapists, occupational therapists, dieticians) who are faced with the need to discuss with their patients topics like eating, exercise, smoking, medication use and drinking. We wrote it because we could not locate a method specifically geared towards behavior change in healthcare settings, where time with the patient is often limited. We have been puzzled by this almost complete absence of attention to the subject of encouraging behavior change, knowing how much time is spent on this activity in healthcare consultations. The problem of poor compliance has been endlessly studied, yet few teachable methods have emerged from this body of research. Our method is geared not only to health promotion consultations, but to the management of many chronic conditions like heart disease and diabetes. It therefore has relevance for both hospital and primary healthcare settings. The method is applicable to any behavior. We believe that certain basic processes operate in any behavior change effort. We all make resolutions to change, and we all know the experience of failure! So too, in trying to help others to change, i.e. our patients, we encounter similar problems in consultations about smoking, drinking, eating and so on. Usually these methods involve some form of direct persuasion or advice-giving. Usually it is a struggle. In developing a different approach we have focused on common underlying principles and methods, at the expense of obvious differences across behaviors.

Why is it not sufficient simply to give patients advice, or 'to educate' them as this activity is sometimes called? Is the kind of method described in this book not unnecessarily complicated? Our starting point is a concern about the limitations of advice-giving, not in general, but in consultations about behavior change, where we have observed frustration among practitioners and patients alike in their response to this approach. Well-meant advice so often seems to slide into unproductive persuasion, disagreement or a blank look from the patient, whose concerns can so easily be overlooked. Practitioners often sense the potential for conflict, and avoid raising the subject of behavior change in the first place. While advice-giving seems to work reasonably well with some patients, sometimes, particularly when there is a good rapport between practitioner and patient, we are concerned about the reliance on this approach as the guiding framework for talk about health behavior change. We believe it is possible to provide the practitioner with a broader, patient-centered framework which is more satisfying to use, more respectful of the uniqueness of each patient and, we suspect, more effective as well. This might be more complicated than simply dispensing advice, but it is probably necessary because the discussion about health behavior change is itself not necessarily a simple matter.

This is a *patient-centered* method, in the sense that patients are given as much opportunity as possible to identify and resolve behavior change issues. It is also *directive*, in the sense that practitioners are encouraged to provide clear structure to the consultation and to raise whatever subject they wish. *Negotiation* is probably the best term to describe this level of interaction (Botehlo, 1992). It is different, for example, from a consultation in which bad news is broken to a patient, or from one in which the practitioner must take clear control of the resolution of a medical problem. Behavior change consultations have a particular edge to them, a sometimes 'itchy' or uncomfortable tension between what the practitioner wants, and the anticipated or actual response of the patient. Our method is an attempt to ensure that this kind of consultation has a humane and respectful quality. Because the patient is encouraged to be as active as possible in making decisions, it should also be more effective than the simpler forms of advice-giving we so often slip into.

We make no apology for unashamedly placing emphasis on the process, in addition to the content, of consultations. It would be much simpler if only the content was significant. It would then be a matter of applying techniques to patients. Unfortunately, such an approach to health behavior change consultations would run into serious trouble. *How* we speak to patients is likely to be just as important as *what* we say to them. This book does not contain important information about specific behaviors and problems. We assume that practitioners have access to expert information in the various specialties (e.g. diet, excessive drinking, smoking), and can integrate this into the method described below, particularly when exchanging information with patients (see Chapter 5).

In theory, practitioners should be able to use the strategies in this book merely by reading about them and then watching carefully what happens in practice. However, such an approach is far from ideal, particularly if the practitioner does not have a reasonable grounding in the patient-centered approach to consulting. The same high standards expected of any professional activity should surely apply here as well. Therefore, training, peer support and ongoing professional development are strongly recommended.

The issue of scientific evidence in this field is an interesting one. A research-conscious reader will wonder whether there is any scientific basis to this method. Attention will probably focus on the *big question*: Does *it* work? The answer is, 'yes, and no'! Some strategies have been evaluated in randomized controlled trials, others not at all. In truth, there is no such thing as *it*, merely a collection of different strategies for use in different situations.

Should one not wait for the outcome of further evaluation before publishing a method of this kind? Our decision not to do this is borne of frustration. Replicable methods simply do not exist. This has led research teams to develop methods which are often poorly described. A statement like, 'Patients were given advice and information about ...', is not uncommon in the description of methods. We believe this approach to be inadequate. More precision is needed about the actual method used, how it was taught to practitioners, and how quality control was maintained throughout the study. We decided to publish this method in order to encourage others to embark on more rigorous evaluation of their work.

The three authors of this book have experience of being scientists, practitioners and trainers. This is not always a comfortable mixture. Scientists we meet challenge us about evidence, and practitioners complain about the narrow preoccupations of science. Some trainees frown at the complexity of methods and others shake their heads about oversimplification. We have thus adopted the role of what Gerard Egan (1994) has called a 'translator', someone who moves between the worlds of theory and practice, trying to bridge the gap between these sometimes distant worlds. Our goal has been to try to cast off jargon, to look for the common ground across theories, and to promote the idea of a generic behavior change method, capable of adaptation to suit the needs of practitioners with different interests and abilities.

We have deliberately not given this approach a name, although for the sake of convenience we do refer to it as a 'method'. To give it a name could lead to misunderstanding. It might be seen as a single entity, as a new and unique method, when in fact it is merely a collection of strategies embedded in a familiar patient-centered framework. It might then be viewed as something which is neatly packaged, ready to be given to patients (or evaluated by researchers) much like one would deliver a dose of intervention or medicine. We would much prefer the boundaries of these strategies to remain loose, so as to encourage adaptation, refinement and the thoughtful development of new strategies.

Some readers will wonder about the links between these strategies and motivational interviewing (Miller & Rollnick 1991). This is discussed in more detail in the final chapter. Briefly, the strategies in this book are all geared towards helping the practitioner approach the 'spirit' of motivational interviewing (Rollnick and Miller 1995), in which resistance is minimized through the use of skilful listening in a constructive discussion about behavior change. This 'spirit' is congruent with the more general use of a patient-centered approach to the consultation (Stewart et al 1995). Some of the strategies in this book emerged directly from early attempts to develop a brief form of motivational interviewing for use in health promotion consultations (Rollnick et al 1992). However, since we cannot expect healthcare practitioners to practice listening skills to a uniformly high standard (something we regret), and because they do not necessarily have the time to explore some of the more personal issues which permeate motivational interviewing sessions, it would be unwise to equate the strategies in this book with motivational interviewing.

A word about terminology, and spelling: with the rapid diffusion of written material across the Atlantic and Pacific Oceans, the differences in spelling conventions between North America and other English-speaking countries was a major problem for us. For instance, the spelling of the word 'behavior' gave rise to much discussion. Put simply, it was possible to follow only one convention, and we have taken the risk of using North American spelling. We can only hope that our readers from Europe and other countries do not feel too offended!

This method is merely a preliminary outline of what should become a more sophisticated approach as ideas and practice develop over the coming years. In this sense, it is a beginning of a process rather than a polished end-product. We hope that practitioners, trainers and researchers will be able to adapt it to suit their needs.

REFERENCES

Botelho R 1992 A negotiation model for the doctor–patient relationship. Family Practice 9:210–218
Egan G 1994 The skilled helper: a problem management approach to helping. Brooks/Cole, Pacific Grove, California
Miller W R, Rollnick S 1991 Motivational interviewing: preparing people to change addictive behavior. The Guilford Press, New York
Rollnick S, Heather N, Bell A 1992 Negotiating behaviour change in medical settings: the development of brief motivational interviewing. Journal of Mental Health 1:25–37
Rollnick S, Miller W R 1995 What is motivational interviewing? Behavioural & Cognitive Psychotherapy 23:325–334
Stewart M, Stewart M, Belle Brown J et al 1995 Patient-centered medicine: transforming the clinical method. Sage Publications, Thousand Oaks

Acknowledgements

Many of the ideas in this book have their origin in the work of William R. Miller, from the University of New Mexico in Albuquerque. His work on motivational interviewing in the addictions field has been inspiring and beyond the bounds of such a brief acknowledgement. Our debt to him is considerable. The work of Jim Prochaska and Carlo DiClemente, who developed the stages of change model, has likewise permeated our teaching, clinical work, and the writing of this book. Some of the strategies outlined in this book emerged from a method which we originally called brief motivational interviewing; we acknowledge the inspiration of our colleague Alison Bell from Sydney, Australia, who helped us develop them.

A number of people afforded us the privilege of looking through a window into their world of work. Professor N.C.H. Stott and colleagues from the Department of General Practice, University of Wales, College of Medicine, provided valuable opportunities to exchange ideas about different kinds of consultations. In particular, the innovative use of the agenda-setting chart in multiple behavior consultations arose directly out of collaborative work with the diabetes research team. Dr Ed Bernstein from the Department of Emergency Medicine, Boston City Hospital kept our feet on the ground with the ultimate challenge: brief intervention while stitching up a stab wound! Entry into the world of cardiac medicine was afforded by the exchange of ideas with Dr Richard Leukar from Albuquerque, New Mexico and Dr Dorian Dugmore from Adidas, UK. Wing Commander Phil Smithson from the Royal Air Force, UK, being a mountaineer, apparently saw little difficulty in changing the ethos and practice of literally hundreds of physical training instructors. Dr David Tappin from the Glasgow Hospital for Sick Children in Scotland, afforded us the privilege of looking into the consultations of midwives, while the Diabetes Research Team at Llandough Hospital in Cardiff, raised a challenge which could keep us busy for a lifetime: if the ethos of the consultation is to change, then so must the design of the treatment system.

Our sincere thanks to Julian Rollnick who meticulously read through chapter drafts, and to Jeff Allison who generated such stimulating discussion about the concepts we were using. Similarly, Carla Hirsh gave us useful feedback about the clarity and usefulness of the material; Lionel Jacobson did a wonderful job of correcting the proofs; Gillian Tober provoked us to reconsider our definition of motivation; and Richard Botelho first set us thinking about the parameters of negotiation in healthcare consultations. Then there was someone from the distant past who stands up like a beacon: Ewart Hood, a psychologist colleague, who left his job in primary health care with a weary look, and the following comment: 'These doctors and nurses, they struggle continuously with behavior change. That's what we should be helping them with.' Finally, our editor at Churchill Livingstone, Alex Mathieson, was kind, efficient and supportive, a master at encouraging behavior change.

PART I

Introduction

OVERVIEW

The aim of this book is to provide some relief from the grip of a paradox: so many patients are passive in the consulting room, yet to succeed with behavior change they need to be active, vigilant decision makers. The origins of this passivity do not lie only within the patients, but also in the way they are spoken to and dealt with by the practitioners. This chapter summarizes a method for encouraging patients to be more active collaborators in talk about behavior change. The next chapter covers some theoretical underpinnings and principles of good practice. In Part II (Chapters 3–5) the method itself is described, while in Part III (Chapters 6–8) attention is focused on practical application, training and other broader issues.

Decisions are made about all kinds of things in healthcare settings, about investigations, interventions, medications, and so on. Different situations demand different responses from the practitioner, some requiring greater control over decision making than others. This book focuses only upon consultations about behavior change where, unfortunately, there are limitations to exerting too much control over decision making: telling patients what to do might be a relatively straightforward procedure, but it might not be the most effective or the most rewarding approach to take with patients. The goal of this book is to promote greater flexibility and skillfulness in the consultation about behavior change.

HEALTH BEHAVIOR CHANGE

The drama of behavior change and resistance to it plays itself out across the full spectrum of daily life. From the willful child resisting a bath to the politician apparently stuck in a destructive conflict, lie a few critical processes: someone, often someone *else*, believes that change is a good idea. One often assumes that the person has the ability to change, if only he or she really wanted to. Conflict and moral judgments are usually close to the surface.

In the consulting room this drama is typically confined to just two people, with the practitioner usually wanting to talk about health behavior change with a patient who might appear to lack motivation. One might think that the practitioner's task, aided by the gravitas of professional authority, would be a fairly straightforward one: advise the patient to eat less, change medication use, take more exercise, drink less alcohol or whatever might be in his or her best interest. Yet this apparently simple exercise in persuasion has bedevilled many a consultation. *Why don't you think about ...* is frequently met with *mmm* from the patient, or a more defiant *Yes, but...*

These consultations have a particular ring to them, a tension about questions like *Why should I change?* and *How can I do it?*, the answers to which seldom imply accord between patient and practitioner. The potential for disagreement rises and falls, but is rarely absent. The atmosphere in behavior change discussions can be quite different from those in which the patient is in a more passive role and feels no responsibility to behave differently; for example, when being relieved of pain by intervention of some kind, or when the subject of discussion is bereavement. Practitioners are usually trying to *persuade* patients in talk about behavior change:

> Practitioner: [taking a deep breath!] *I wonder whether it might be useful to think about taking just a little less fatty food over the next few months?*

> Patient: *I don't overdo it really. Occasionally it gets a bit out of hand, when I'm under stress, but mostly, I'm very controlled.*

> Practitioner: *It will certainly help with your heart.*

> Patient: *Yes, I see what you mean, but...*

This breakdown in communication can arise because the patient does not view the change as important, or because he or she does not feel confident about succeeding. Thus far, it is apparently the patient's problem. However, resistance can also arise because of the way the patient is being spoken to. The culprit, we believe, is usually the use of direct persuasion by the practitioner, which increases the potential for disagreement.

Practitioners have different ways of coping with this situation. Some effectively give up: *There's no point in trying too hard, because these patients don't really want to change their lifestyles.* Blaming the patient is just one way of dealing with resistance. Some just keep going, give the advice, apparently discharge their duty, and move on to the next patient. Others confine their attention only to those who really want to change.

This book examines routes out of this impasse, in pursuit of creative consulting methods in which the patient is encouraged to be the expert about behavior change. One might argue that this is simply good healthcare practice, that it involves little more than the use of a respectful, patient-centered consulting style, and that there is no need to develop concepts and strategies specific to the subject of behavior change. Our view is that the tension about the why and how of change, so prevalent in these consultations, makes it a subject worthy of study in its own right, capable of generating new ways of tackling familiar problems.

Some readers might observe that using alternatives to direct persuasion and empowering the patient has clear parallels in good behavior change practice at home, in schools or in business meetings. This might be the case. We hesitate to generalize, however, because these wider encounters might be governed by different dynamics and ethical principles. Our focus is on the healthcare consultation.

COMMON CONCERNS, CONDITIONS AND COMPLAINTS

The method described in this book is potentially applicable to any behavior change consultation in a healthcare setting:

In the hospital we can work on our side of the problem – regular monitoring, advice about self-care, treatment when it's needed, but she must work on her side of the problem as well – lose weight, get more exercise and stop smoking before it kills her. The problem is this: she listens, but she never does anything. (Doctor, aged 56, outpatient clinic)

I try to advise them about diet. Every day I do this. Information, leaflets, diaries to fill in and lengthy discussions here in the clinic. It's not an easy job. Nice people, most of them, but hopeless at making changes. (Dietician, aged 24, community health centre)

He must know it is a problem. I mean he can't walk too far, he is so short of breath. Yet will he admit it? Will he talk about doing something about it? (Nurse, aged 27, hospital ward)

He comes to see me regularly, we talk about his drinking and what it is doing to his life. He makes his promises, and he breaks his promises, again and again. Sometimes I feel like screaming at him and giving him an ultimatum. (Health promotion counselor, aged 40, primary care clinic)

Among the most frequently encountered *changes in behavior* which practitioners focus on are:

- eat less, eat different things, adjust timing of meals
- drink less alcohol, abstain altogether
- be more physically active, do particular exercises
- smoke fewer cigarettes, abstain altogether
- take a new medication, a different one, replace one with another, at a different time
- monitor levels of glucose in the blood, ingest more/less liquid
- reduce intake of a substance, abstain altogether.

Consultations about these changes occur in a wide range of *patients* who are, or who are thought to be:

- at risk of suffering from heart disease
- recovering from a heart attack
- diabetic
- overweight or obese
- pregnant
- at risk of contracting sexually transmitted diseases
- chronic pain sufferers
- problem drinkers

- substance misusers
- asthmatic.

The *practitioners* involved are usually:

- doctors
- nurses
- nutritionists
- dietitians
- physiotherapists
- health visitors
- health promotion practitioners
- psychologists and psychiatrists
- counselors
- health educators
- fitness instructors
- dentists.

The *settings* in which patients are seen are thus widespread:

- primary care
- inpatient
- outpatient
- community health projects
- emergency room
- leisure facilities
- occupational health clinics.

It is obvious from these lists that we are not just referring to health promotion consultations among relatively well populations. The management of chronic problems like diabetes, heart disease and obesity all involve attempts to encourage behavior change. These consultations occur in hospital inpatient and outpatient settings, as well as community-based clinics and health centers.

BEHAVIOR CHANGE: WHOSE PROBLEM IS IT?

The logic with which the patient can be viewed as responsible for the outcome of a behavior change consultation has a formidable ring to it: after all, it is not the practitioners who need to change their behavior, is it? One can quite easily rationalize the process thus: *What you* [the patient] *put in, is what you get out*. This can take an aggressive form: *I can't help these people if they don't want to help themselves ...* ; or it can reflect a genuine desire not to impose one's values and will on the patient:

I'll help them if they want help, but if they don't, that's fine. ... I respect the person more than I respect my right to tell them what to do. (Primary care physician, aged 41)

Whatever our approach to behavior change, two things are fairly certain: the discussion about change with patients never goes away, and the outcome of the consultation is affected by our consulting behavior. There is a lot that can be done to make matters worse, or better. Behavior change, or the lack of it, is not just the patient's problem.

Practitioner makes matters worse

Practitioner: *Have you thought about losing some weight?*

Patient: *Yes, many times, but I can't seem to manage. It's my one comfort, my eggs in the morning, my fried chicken at lunch. I'm stuck in the house so much these days.*

Practitioner: *It would certainly help your blood pressure.*

Patient: *I know, but what do I do when I really want my two eggs for breakfast? It's a tradition in our family. [Sighs] I always get told to lose weight when I come to this clinic.*

Practitioner: *Have you thought about a gradual approach, like leaving out just one of the eggs for a while, and seeing what a difference it makes?*

Patient: *Yes but, what sort of difference will this make?*

Practitioner: *Over time, as you succeed with one thing, you can try another, and gradually your weight will come down.*

Patient: *Not in my house. The temptations are everywhere, you should just see what's on the table to munch, any time you want.*

Practitioner: *Have you talked to your partner about leaving these off the table, just to make it easier for you?*

Patient: *Yes, but…*

Practitioner makes matters better

Practitioner: *Have you thought·about losing some weight?*

Patient: *Yes, many times, but I can't seem to manage. It's my one comfort, my eggs in the morning, my fried chicken at lunch. I'm stuck in the house so much these days.*

Practitioner: *It's not easy.*

Patient: *Say that again!*

Practitioner: *Some people prefer to change their eating, others to get more exercise. Both can help with losing weight. How do you really feel at the moment?*

Patient: *I'm not sure. I always get told to lose weight when I come to this clinic.*

Practitioner: *It's like we always know what's good for you, as if it's just a matter of going out there, and one, two, three, and you lose weight!*

Patient: *Exactly. I'm not sure I can change my eating right now. I used to get a lot more exercise, but life's changed and I've got lazy.*

Practitioner: *Well, I'm certainly not here to harangue you. In fact, all I want to do is understand how you really feel, and whether there is some way you can keep your blood pressure down. Perhaps there isn't at the moment?*

Patient: *Well, I could think about…*

When patients fail to endorse practitioners' seemingly rational, friendly and helpful advice, it is understandable that practitioners should feel frustrated, or even blame the patients for irrational obstinacy. Indeed, a large body of research on compliance also appears to have embraced the notion that lack of success is basically a patient resistance problem (Butler et al 1996). According to this model, the practitioner's role is to communicate information clearly, on the assumption that expert knowledge needs to be understood by the more or less passive and ignorant patients. But the problem is not that simple, and patient resistance is not just a result of poor information delivery.

It is quite possible that expert knowledge has a limited role in behavior change discussion. For example, in the above dialog, there was talk about blood pressure, but it appeared that the patient knew about this anyway. Like it or not, the practitioner soon moves from the world of specialist knowledge into the realm of encouragement and looking at options for change. How this is handled is critical to the outcome of the consultation. If resistance arises, and behavior change is not seriously considered by the patient in the consultation, the practitioner could well bear equal responsibility for this. If there is a specialist skill in the behavior change field it is in the artful handling of this interchange, whatever the health behavior or pathology under discussion.

TRADITIONAL METHODS AND TRAINING

The choice of advice-giving as the strategy for encouraging behavior change has its origins in so many aspects of everyday life. How else do you do it? If you want a child to wash, and you decide not simply to issue an order, you try to explain why this would be a good idea. If you want to put an intravenous line into a patient in pain, you do the same thing. You provide factual information and good reasons for your course of action. Using this strategy in behavior consultations seems a perfectly logical approach. For example:

> I think your back pain is made much worse by all the weight you are carrying so I'm giving you this diet sheet which I would like you to follow. Let's set a target of you losing 30 pounds over the next 6 months. I'm sure this will take some of the strain off your back.

This approach is heavily reinforced in the general education of practitioners. Treating patients carries the assumption that expert knowledge is required, and advice-giving is merely seen as the device for delivering this knowledge. Being effective in the management of so many kinds of problems, this device is then quite understandably used in consultations about behavior change.

If practitioners do receive specific training in dealing with health behavior change, it is usually in the acquisition of ever more sophisticated specialist knowledge about different problems, at the expense of looking at methods of communicating with patients. They might receive educational input on excessive drinking, diabetes, smoking or asthma, but they seldom discuss the communication challenges that arise in all of these consultations, whatever the topic of conversation might be.

Given this approach to training, one might imagine that there is a lack of theory and research on the more general subject of behavior change, yet there is a considerable amount. Journals in psychology and in healthcare are not short of ideas and research on behavior change, yet few attempts are made to bridge the gulf between theory and practice. Rather, general principles of behavior change have become submerged in the paraphernalia of specialist expertise. Our goal is to demonstrate that there are exciting concepts and methods which can be brought to bear on any behavior change discussion, and that this is a subject worthy of study in the training of practitioners.

WHERE IS THE MAGIC BULLET?

There is no magic bullet. Indeed, our conclusion is that to improve matters, our models and methods need to become a little more sophisticated. We should move away from the notion that giving advice will suffice. This does not mean that every behavior change consultation will be an enormous time-consuming effort. Sometimes it might take a little longer, but not always. In the dialog presented on page 7, the more productive consultation was more artful, but not more time consuming. In general, however, there are no simple solutions to helping people with behavior change, and if you are looking for a magic bullet, then think about another professional activity!

THE METHOD

After spending many years training practitioners and counselors, and discussing behavior change with our own patients, a collection of strategies emerged which could be applied to any brief behavior change consultation. Our goals were to provide practitioners with a useful framework, to improve the quality of their training, and to encourage the evaluation of methods for promoting behavior change.

Origins

The method was developed over a 10-year period, in which ideas and strategies were tried out in real and simulated consultations. Some of the strategies emerged from a study of health promotion among excessive drinkers in a general hospital setting, which led to the development of a method called 'brief motivational interviewing' (Rollnick et al 1992). Others emerged from work with smokers (Rollnick et al 1997, Butler et al, in press) and people with diabetes (Stott et al 1995, 1996). Equally important were our experiences in the training of doctors, nurses and dietitians, in which behavior change problems were examined in simulated encounters and then tried out in everyday practice.

The method outlined here comes from two broad sources: on the one hand, developments in the addictions field like motivational interviewing (Miller 1983, Miller & Rollnick 1991) and the stages of change model (DiClemente & Prochaska 1998); and on the other hand, the patient-centered approach to the consultation (Stewart et al 1995). The method leans heavily on these innovations, particularly those from the addictions field, and in this sense it is by no means original. Rather, it is an attempt to refine and adapt these ideas and techniques, for use in a brief patient-centered consultation.

Refinement of specialist addiction methods was necessary because one cannot expect practitioners in healthcare settings, who have so many other priorities, to use the often complex and time-consuming methods employed by specialists in the addictions field. Adaptation was also necessary in order to embrace what is far more common in general healthcare consultations than in specialist settings: while specialists often focus on a particular behavioral topic in relatively greater depth, generalists typically encounter a broader range of interrelated problems and behaviors. They are closer, particularly in primary care, to the ever-shifting world of personal and social circumstances, and they are aware of the subtle ways in which one health behavior affects another. The patient-centered method forms an essential framework for understanding this context. Thus, the behavior change strategies described in this book are embedded in a framework for working with the 'whole' person. They are not magic bullets, but ways of structuring a conversation which maximize the individual's freedom to talk and to think about change in an atmosphere free of coercion and the provision of premature solutions.

A collection of strategies

This book contains something more like a framework, or a collection of strategies, than a discrete method. The 'how to do it' chapters (3, 4 and 5) in Part II follow a sequential journey through a consultation in which a number of key *tasks* are pinpointed (raising the subject, setting an agenda, and so on). We emphasize the practitioner's freedom to choose a task which most suits the patient. Setting an agenda, for example, will be essential with some patients, and irrelevant to others.

There is obviously no single way of carrying out a particular task. We have called the different ways of carrying out a task *strategies*. Thus, within most of the tasks described in Part II a selection of strategies is described. Practitioners are free to choose the one that most suits the situation in which they find themselves.

For the sake of simplicity we have taken the liberty of using the term 'method' in this book. However, we have deliberately not given this method a name, to avoid creating the misleading impression that behavior change consultations involve doing *a*, then *b*, followed by *c*. Similarly, while we have identified a sequence of tasks to be used in different parts of a consultation, our aim is to provide a menu of options for practitioners to choose from. Consultations more often go around in circles or cycles than following a simple linear path. Our hope is that the tasks and strategies give some sense of direction to this activity.

OVERVIEW

Figure 1.1 provides an outline of the key tasks which are discussed in detail in Part II (Chapters 3, 4 and 5). Two obvious initial tasks are to *establish rapport* and to *set an agenda* (Chapter 3). The latter is sometimes not necessary, because practitioner and patient know what it is they wish to talk about. At other times it is essential and often complex. We have distinguished between single and multiple behavior consultations, the latter involving a delicate negotiation about what to talk about, for example, smoking, eating, exercise or some other personal concern.

Having agreed to discuss a particular change in behaviour, the goal is to understand exactly how the patient feels about this. The task *assess*

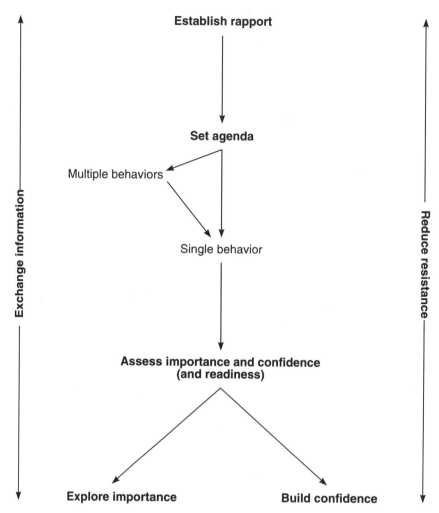

Figure 1.1　Key tasks in consultations about behavior change.

importance and confidence is designed to achieve this (Chapter 3). Some patients need more time to *explore the importance* of change. Others are already convinced that they should change, and they want to, but need help to *build confidence* in their ability to achieve this. These are the next two tasks (Chapter 4). When they are completed the next step will become clearer. It may be one of further exploration and discussion or it may be planning the first step of an action plan.

There are two tasks which run right through the consultation process. These are *exchanging information* and *reducing resistance* (Chapter 5). Exchanging information will be used at various points to ensure that both practitioner and patient fully understand the key issues and each other's viewpoint. The patient might at any time show reluctance, defensiveness or some other suggestion of resistance. This is an indication that all is not well in the consultation, and it might be necessary to change tack in some way, change the pace of the consultation or discuss this with the patient. All of these tasks are described in detail in Part II, where we identify strategies that we have found useful to help the process along.

HOW TO USE THIS BOOK

How much time do you have?

The method is designed to enable practitioners to penetrate behavior change consultation tasks to varying degrees of depth. For example:

Just a few hours

Absorb the 'spirit' of the method (see Chapters 1 and 2), and familiarize yourself with some of the *tasks* identified in the single-page outline in Figure 1.1. Identify the most useful ones, and take note of some of the *useful questions* you might use in your consultations. These are listed at the beginning of each chapter in Part II. Are you familiar with any of the typical clinical encounters described in Chapter 6? If so, these accounts will also give you a good idea of the overall spirit of the method.

About a day

In addition to understanding the most suitable *tasks*, absorb some of the *useful questions* which are associated with each task. You should have time to explore some of the detailed strategies and visual aids associated with each task. Discussion with colleagues, preferably using simulated patients for practice, will help a lot.

More than a day

With this amount of time you should be able to examine and practice the *strategies* embedded within the tasks. Practice these with simulated or real patients, and return to the book for clarification and further reading.

What skills do you have?

If you are reasonably familiar with the practice of using listening skills (e.g. open questions, summarizing, reflective listening), you should have no difficulty in learning to use the more directive strategies in this book. If not, we strongly recommend that you work on this aspect of the method first, since this is the fuel that drives a quality behavior change consultation. We are not saying, however, that you need to be an experienced counselor in order to succeed.

Creative adaptation, not slavish adoption

The collection of strategies in Part II are written out in a concrete form. The aim is to provide practitioners with a clear vision of what can work well. We certainly do not mean to imply that this is the only way, or the best way, to proceed. Our goal can be described thus: try it this way, because it will help you get the feel of how to avoid reinforcing resistance and develop the discussion in a constructive way. When you feel more comfortable, adapt the strategy, and make up new ones that suit you and your patients. The context of your work might require considerable adaptation, in which case your collection will contain quite different strategies.

Some practitioners might want to integrate behavior change work into their everyday practice. Others might want to work on a particular project and develop a specific intervention, for example, for people with diabetes, obesity, heart disease or nicotine dependence, or for improving adherence to medication more generally. The breadth of the method described in Part II demands pilot work, practice and refinement. This should not be seen as a problem, but as an opportunity to understand what is going on in your behavior change consultations. To seek clarity, try new ideas, become confused, and have discussions with others are activities that mirror what we would like patients to do. This is no coincidence, because to develop new ways of consulting involves changes in our own behavior. The evidence about practitioner behavior change points clearly to the need for piloting and practice, whether this be in the use of new guidelines or in developing patient-centered consulting methods. A method adapted and refined in-house by you will be more useful than one handed down to you from a book, a trainer or a manager.

REFERENCES

Butler C C, Rollnick S, Stott N C H 1996 The practitioner, the patient and resistance to change: recent ideas on compliance. Canadian Medical Association Journal 154:1357–1362
Butler C C, Rollnick S, Cohen D, Russell I, Bachmann M, Stott N (in press) Motivational consulting versus brief advice for smokers in general practice: a randomised trial. British Journal of General Practice
DiClemente C C, Prochaska J 1998 Toward a comprehensive, transtheoretical model of change: stages of change and addictive behaviors. In: Miller W R, Heather N (eds) Treating addictive behaviors, 2nd edn. Plenum, New York
Miller W R 1983 Motivational interviewing with problem drinkers. Behavioural Psychotherapy 1:147–172
Miller W R, Rollnick S 1991 Motivational interviewing: preparing people to change addictive behavior. Guilford Press, New York

Rollnick S, Butler C C, Stott N 1997 Helping smokers make decisions: the enhancement of brief intervention for general medical practice. Patient Education and Counseling 31:191–203

Rollnick S, Heather N, Bell A 1992 Negotiating behaviour change in medical settings: the development of brief motivational interviewing. Journal of Mental Health 1:25–37

Stewart M, Stewart M, Belle Brown J et al 1995 Patient-centered medicine. Transforming the clinical method. Sage, Thousand Oaks

Stott N C H, Rollnick S, Rees M, Pill R 1995 Innovation in clinical method: diabetes care and negotiating skills. Family Practice 12:413–418

Stott N C H, Rees M, Rollnick S, Pill R, Hackett P 1996 Professional responses to innovation in clinical method: diabetes care and negotiation skills. Patient Education and Counseling 29:67–73

2

Foundations: theory and practice

It has been said, apparently since Ancient Greek times, that the three basic tools of medicine are 'the herb', 'the knife' and 'the word' (Grant 1995). This chapter is about the use of 'the word' in behavior change consultations.

A lot has been written about good general consulting skills, much of which is clearly relevant to talking about behavior change. However, the behavior change consultation presents some unique challenges which make it quite different from, for example, the breaking of bad news to a patient, or the eliciting of a history of presenting symptoms. Our starting point is that there is a need to study behavior change as a topic in its own right. Our hope is that teachable skills can emerge from this endeavor, that research protocols and educational curricula reflect the importance of this subject, and that these common consultations can be dealt with in a more sophisticated and sensitive manner.

This aim of this chapter is to describe the principles upon which the strategies described in Part II are based. To begin with, we review concepts like readiness, importance and confidence, which provide the theoretical base of the method. Attention will then turn to general guidelines for good practice. Here we will present the case for combining a *patient-centered* with a more *directive* approach to behavior change consultations. A more detailed discussion of theoretical and clinical issues is contained in the final chapter of the book.

THE THEORETICAL BASE: READINESS, IMPORTANCE AND CONFIDENCE

Some themes stood out very clearly from our review of the literature on health psychology and behavior change. First, the idea of *readiness*, derived from the stages of change model (Prochaska & DiClemente 1983, 1986, DiClemente & Prochaska 1998) was a useful starting point for understanding motivation and how best to work with patients. They are not an homogenous group when it comes to behavior change; depending on their degree of readiness to change, they have different needs and should be treated accordingly.

Second, standing out from the different models of behavior change, many of them overlapping and in apparent conflict with one another, were two concepts, *importance* and *confidence*, which helped to explain a patient's degree of motivation or readiness to change. They appeared in different guises in different models, but seemed to point to the same conclusion: if a change feels *important* to you, and you have the *confidence* to achieve it, you will feel more *ready* to have a go, and more likely to succeed. When you are sitting in front of patients, understanding their feelings about these three topics will take you to the heart of the complex forces which surround the topic of behavior change.

Readiness

This is a state of mind which reflects the outcome of quite a lot of psychological activity. For example, one difference between a child who refuses to go to school, another who dithers on the doorstep and a third who leaps enthusiastically onto the school bus is clear-cut: they differ in their readiness. Looking at how this state of mind varies in our work with patients is a useful starting point. Of course, we will want to know *why*, in the above example and many others like it, differences in readiness arise. The concepts of importance and confidence should help with this task. To begin with, however, we have been struck, like many other practitioners, by the value of simply being aware of this fluctuating and sometimes conflict-ridden state of mind, readiness. It has clear implications for how we speak to people, whatever debate there might be about other aspects of the stages of change model (Davidson 1998, Prochaska & DiClemente 1998) (see Chapter 8).

The stages of change model is an attempt to describe readiness and how people move towards making decisions and behavior change in their everyday lives. Its emergence in the field of health promotion and behavior change, which one commentator described as akin to the discovery of a new planet in astronomy (Stockwell 1992), clearly struck a chord with practitioners and researchers alike. People, whether they be patients, practitioners or the public at large, were described as moving through a series of stages when trying to change behavior, from precontemplation through to action and maintenance, along the lines illustrated in Figure 2.1. A thorough attempt was also made to describe the process needed to move from one stage to the next and the therapeutic techniques likely to engage these processes. An updated overview and critique of this model can be found in Miller & Heather (1998).

If we take the example of smoking, which was used in much of the research on this model, someone in the precontemplation stage will think and feel quite differently from someone in the preparation stage. While the former will not actively be thinking about stopping smoking, the latter will be planning very actively. Between these two people lies the person in the contemplation stage, who thinks about stopping, wants to do something about it, but also does not. Most smokers seem to fall into this stage. The

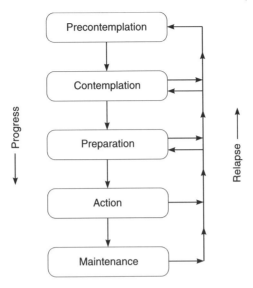

Figure 2.1   The stages of change model.

model states that people are likely to move through these stages in the cyclical manner depicted in Figure 2.1.

This model describes what happens to people as they change in everyday life. If we turn our attention, as the authors have done, to how one helps people who vary in their states of readiness, the usefulness of the model is striking: people have different needs and they do not all need the same kind of help. Unfortunately, too many services have been action oriented, revolving around the small percentage of people who are ready to come forward and take action, typically less than 20% (DiClemente & Prochaska 1998). The appeal of this model to practitioners probably does not lie in the precise definition of stages or the intricacies of stage-specific interventions, but in the provision of general guidance; for example, if someone is not ready to change, action talk will be counterproductive. If this observation of the reason for its popularity is correct (see Rollnick 1998), then unresolved issues like whether stages exist and how to match interventions to stages (discussed in Chapter 8) might not be critically important for present purposes. The model provides a unifying concept, readiness to change, which is so clearly relevant to everyday practice that we should be able to use it as a platform for a behavior change method.

One simple way of using this model in everyday practice, illustrated in Figure 2.2, is to think of a patient's readiness on a continuum, bearing in mind that it is not the patient in general who is more or less ready, but his or her readiness to *make a specific change in behavior.*

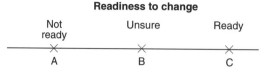

Figure 2.2   A readiness to change continuum.

Patients' needs vary depending on where they lie on this hypothetical continuum. Individuals at A, B and C will talk about quite different things. Some practitioners have even described them as 'different voices' or 'different languages'. The challenge for practitioners then, is to maintain parity or *congruence* with the readiness to change of the individual. This is what we mean by *matching* in this book, although the term has been used in other ways (see Chapter 8).

One can turn this discussion of matching upside-down and ask what happens when you fail to achieve congruence, when you talk in a way which is not suited to the readiness of your patient? If you talk to patient A in Figure 2.2 who is not thinking about change *as if* she was or should be at point C, ready for action and keen to get as much help as possible, you will encounter *resistance*. Jumping ahead of the patient's readiness can be a risky activity.

The stages of change model, with its call to pay attention to these matters, challenges us to think about how we might match the topic of conversation to the readiness to change of the patient. It was this challenge which led us to experiment with different topics in our consultations and to review the literature on health psychology. These activities were stimulated by the question, *why* does a person place him- or herself at a particular point on the readiness continuum? We were relieved to find some common ground between the world of theory and our clinical experience: people's feelings about whether change was worthwhile (importance) and whether they could achieve it (confidence) contributed to our understanding of readiness.

Importance and confidence

In experimental consultations with smokers we asked them why they placed themselves at a given point on a readiness continuum, and two themes repeatedly emerged, reflecting the issues of importance and confidence (Rollnick et al 1997). In fact, we even came across two smokers who placed themselves at around the same place on the continuum, who gave us very different answers to the question 'why do you feel this way?'. They both described themselves as midway along a readiness continuum; one, an elderly man who was very ill with a smoking-related disease, said he was desperate to stop, it was very important to him, but he lacked the con-

---

Box 2.1   Three topics in talk about behavior change

Importance	Confidence	Readiness
Why?	**How? What?**	**When?**
Is it worthwhile?	Can I?	Should I do it now?
Why should I?	How will I do it?	What about other priorities?
How will I benefit?	How will I cope with x, y	
What will change?	and z?	
At what cost?	Will I succeed if... ?	
Do I really want to?	What change... ?	
Will it make a difference?		

---

fidence to succeed; the other said that it was not very important to her to quit, but she had no doubt about her ability to succeed, if she chose to quit smoking. Neither person was ready to stop, both being unsure about it all, but each for completely different reasons. We then found that the themes of readiness, importance and confidence echoed through conversations with people about changes in eating, exercise, drinking and even compulsive shopping.

Box 2.1 lists the kind of questions people might ask themselves about readiness, importance and confidence. How to talk about these questions in a constructive way is our primary objective in this book. The terms readiness, importance and confidence are merely the keys which open the door to these discussions.

Our decision to use the terms *importance* and *confidence* instead of the numerous alternatives available was driven partly by a desire to pursue simplicity of expression, to free practitioners from the weight of jargon which so bedevils some of the literature on behavior change. When it came to the term *importance*, we could have used alternatives like the *pros and cons of change*, or the perceived *costs* and *benefits* of change. However, we wanted to avoid the potentially misleading impression that weighing up the value of change is a matter of balancing the rational components of something akin to a psychological ledger. It can be that simple sometimes, but this weighing up can also be influenced strongly by feelings about other matters beyond the behavior in question, often linked to fundamental values about health and well-being; hence our emphasis on the word importance.

For example, a person who is very overweight might feel that food is a comfort in the face of a difficult life in which well-being is undermined by a host of other problems. The *importance* of a change in eating or exercise behavior is weighed up against the importance of change in other, sometimes more important matters such as saving money by buying cheap food, or being around and attentive to the children in the evenings, rather than going to a gym. This can be a difficult area to talk about, particularly if time is short. Another example comes from the world of chronic disease

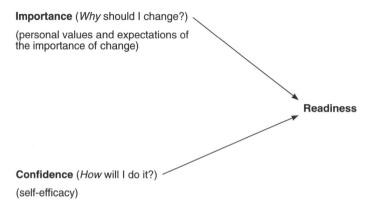

Figure 2.3   The ingredients of readiness to change.

management. Many patients do not feel that they have a labeled condition like diabetes or asthma in the first place. This will obviously affect their feelings about the importance of changes in health behavior. Under these circumstances, value conflict with the practitioner is not uncommon. For example, a practitioner might feel that it is very important to look after one's health and prevent the onset of diseases by adjusting one's lifestyle. Many patients, however, feel otherwise, for a range of reasons. These differences in values will influence beliefs about health and illness, attitudes towards scientific evidence, and the perceived importance of a change in behavior. We chose the term *confidence* instead of *ability* because it focuses on the person's underlying psychological state, and avoids the mistake of assuming that talking about this topic is merely a matter of focusing on 'technical' coping skills.

Figure 2.3 describes one way of viewing the links between these three terms, in which the patient's feelings about importance and confidence contribute to the more general state of readiness to change. These three concepts have a reasonably solid base in psychological theory. A review of the literature on behavior change, in the addictions field and in health psychology, reveals a clear tendency for discussion to revolve around these concepts, particularly importance and confidence (see Chapter 8 for a fuller discussion).

The separation of importance and confidence in Figure 2.3 should not be misunderstood: sometimes the distinction between them is clear; at other times they seem to influence one another. For example, low levels of confidence can often affect a person's feelings and thoughts about the importance of a given change. Someone who has repeatedly failed to maintain abstinence from smoking (i.e. low confidence level) may come to resent the pressures from others to quit, begin to question the validity of health messages, seize on stories of healthy, aged smokers, and come to regard quitting as not worthwhile. Despite this complexity, we believe the distinctions are nevertheless clinically useful. Try talking about confidence when the patient is more concerned with the value or importance of change, and the outcome will be a quite serious mismatch.

The method described in Part II is based on a framework in which monitoring readiness is viewed as an ongoing background task in the consultation, with the assessment of importance and confidence forming a platform for constructive talk about change.

Motivation

This is a well-used phrase in consulting rooms, training workshops and the literature on behavior change. Our use of it in this book follows an example set by others, which equates motivation to a person's expressed degree of readiness to change (see Miller & Rollnick 1991). Anything a patient does to enhance his or her sense of either importance or confidence will increase his or her motivation to change. People can thus have motivational problems in the consultation because they do not feel that change is important and/or they are concerned about their ability to achieve it. Building motivation, then, is not just restricted to the importance dimension, a view quite commonly expressed by practitioners and trainers.

Resistance

This is usually viewed as a patient problem. Much of the writing on psychotherapy is based on the assumption that the patient brings resistance into the consulting room. We use the term to refer to an observable pattern of behavior (denial, arguing, putting up objections, showing reluctance to engage in conversation) which is not just a result of what patients bring into the consultation, but also something that is influenced by the way in which practitioners speak to them (Miller & Rollnick 1991). Use a confrontational interviewing style and resistance will increase; assume greater readiness to change than is the case, by talking about action when the patient is not ready for this, and the resistance that emerges will be at least partly the responsibility of the practitioner.

By thinking of resistance as an interpersonal problem which the practitioner can enhance or diminish, we do not mean to imply that the patient is merely a hapless victim of insensitive consulting. People struggling with behavior change go through their own internal battles, between indulgence and restraint (e.g. gambling, smoking, eating), and between carrying on as usual or initiating a new activity (exercise, a new medication). Sometimes this involves conflict with others who place pressure on them to change. Sometimes people come into the consulting room expecting or fearing that these struggles will be exposed. Insensitive consulting can elicit and reinforce this resistance. Good consulting involves allowing the person to express his or her fears about change, without being made to feel judged or pressurized into action. This topic is taken up in greater detail in Chapter 5.

GUIDELINES FOR GOOD PRACTICE

Constructive talk about topics like readiness, importance and confidence requires some structure to be provided by the practitioner (i.e. a *directive process*), and some ability to listen and follow what is being said (i.e. a *patient-centered process*). The remainder of this chapter focuses on the general principles of consulting about behavior change, which are as important, if not more so, than the detailed step-by-step guidelines in the following three chapters. Like learning to dance, if one focuses too much on detailed steps, one can lose awareness of the overall gestalt or 'spirit' of the activity.

We balk at the view of the consultation in which the practitioner is seen as providing a dose of this or that intervention to the patient. There has been a tendency to view the stages of change model in this way. It might be a useful starting point, but quite soon the practitioner will be left with the task of responding to the ever shifting world of behavior change talk where finer skills and sensitivities will be required. We start with the topic of advice-giving, which, unfortunately, is all too often based on the principle of handing down expertise to the passive patient.

What's wrong with advice-giving?

A 55-year-old man had been suffering from insulin-dependent diabetes since the age of 11 years, and had tried to live his life 'despite' his disease, even to the point of ignoring the need to properly monitor his blood glucose levels. This had severely affected his health. He was no longer able to feel his legs, and had difficulty walking. He had been advised, many dozens of times, to monitor his glucose levels, look after his diet, get more exercise, and so on. In fact, he could have written a leaflet on good practice in diabetic care! But he made little effort to look after himself. Then one day a doctor and nurse decided to take a different approach. No more attention would be paid to health behavior change in the consultation; they were going to find out what was important to him, and how he felt about the disease. The rapport between them and the patient improved over a number of months. It emerged that he did not feel that it was possible or worthwhile to look after himself. He later described the doctor and nurse as having 'brought me into the real world'. His monitoring of blood glucose improved.

If advice-giving was sufficient to encourage behavior change there would be no need to write this book. While this sometimes has its place in consultations about behavior change, particularly the process of providing information to patients, our concern is that it should not provide the dominant framework for teaching and practice (Rollnick et al 1993). The above story about one of our patients illustrates the limitations of repeated advice-giving. While the more recent discussions with the nurse–doctor team had taken a little more time than their average consultation, many, many dozens of fruitless hours, over three decades, had been spent on persuading this man to look after himself.

We do not mean to imply that advice-giving should be discarded. It would be unwise to be either flippant or dismissive about a consulting style which is so easy to learn and use. Advice-giving is appropriately entrenched in many aspects of healthcare. Our comments here refer only to consultations about health behavior change, where it is easy for nursing or medical students to absorb the familiar *modus operandi* and develop advice-giving as a consulting habit. This can be done with compassion and clarity, and there is no doubt that it can be effective. One of us has a sporting team mate who immortalized the value of advice-giving. He went to the doctor with a sports injury and came hobbling back to the next game, free of cigarettes for the first time in his adult life. 'Yes,' he said, 'I went to the doc, and he gave me a hard time. He lifted his finger and said, "watch it, stop smoking, OK?". So I've done it, and that's it, end of story'. Some 3 years later this man remained free of nicotine dependence. We cannot be sure that this is exactly what the doctor said to him, or what his state of readiness to change was at the time. Nevertheless, advice it certainly was.

There is evidence which shows that simple advice can effect behavior change, perhaps more so in the fields of smoking and excessive drinking than eating or exercise (see, for example, Ashenden et al 1997). Our concerns are that only a small proportion of recipients respond, that it renders patients passive in the consultation and that giving advice can lead to the threat of disagreement in talk about behavior change.

Consider this response from a research interview with a Scottish mother in a study of the work of health visitors by McIntosh:

She keeps tellin' me, 'Do this, do that.' It makes ye feel like a moron, that yer no capable o' lookin' after yer baby. … Ah always feel guilty after she's been as if ah've been doin' everything wrong. It makes me mad. Ah don't say anything at the time, ah just mutter a few oaths when she's gone. (McIntosh 1986 p. 26. In Heritage & Sefi 1992 p. 410)

Advice-giving has been defined as a sequence in a consultation in which the practitioner *describes, recommends or forwards a preferred course of action* (Heritage & Sefi 1992). Analysis of consultations reveals that requests for advice from patients are relatively rare (Heritage & Sefi 1992, Silverman 1997). In the case of Scottish health visitors, the majority of the advice sequences were delivered by them to patients in 'strongly prescriptive terms', which emerge in the form of *overt recommendations*, often couched in the *imperative mood* ('… be very very quiet at night …') and using *verbs of obligation* ('you should …', 'you ought to …') (Heritage & Sefi 1992).

Advice-giving has the appearance of simplicity: just give people information and tell them what to do or how to do it. In practice, however, it is far from simple. Practitioners have to keep a firm eye on the clock and avoid a disagreement and communication breakdown. Silverman (1997) describes a number of ways in which HIV counselors avoid being too personal when giving advice, for fear of being met with outright rejection from the patient: they couch their advice as if it is information, something he called the 'Advice as Information Sequence'; they also use the word *if* so as to give the patient freedom to turn down the advice; and they make oblique references to other people when delivering advice, for example, *What we say in this clinic is …* Thus advice-giving is not straightforward. Its passage is often delicately steered to avoid outright rejection by the patient.

Our hunch is that advice-giving consists of at least two elements which are worth teasing out. First, there is the process of providing the patient with information. This crucial part of consulting cannot be dispensed with. Our concern is about the way in which this is done. As commonly practiced, this activity can render the patient a passive recipient of expert knowledge, and too often takes the form of a single verbal intervention combined with arguments for change. Fear induction is often part of this process. For example, *Your blood sugar readings suggest that you have been slipping a bit recently, and that you should now be working a bit harder on bringing this under control.* We believe that the study of information-giving and recent developments in motivational interviewing provide a clear and teachable approach to information exchange which maximizes patient autonomy and is more likely to enhance patients' motivation to change. This is discussed in detail in Chapter 5, where a three-step sequence (elicit–provide–elicit) for information exchange is described.

A second component of advice-giving is persuasion: telling patients what you think they should do, or how they should do it. This is where the chief limitation of advice-giving lies. Telling patients what they should do can frequently undermine their autonomy and generate resistance. Here is a typical example of the kind of *'yes, but …'* dialog which results from advice-giving.

Practitioner: *You need to reduce the fat in your diet. You should try to avoid fried food, for a start.*

Patient: *But the kids won't eat anything if it doesn't come with chips.*

Practitioner: *Well, chips aren't very good for them either, perhaps you could all eat more rice or pasta dishes.*

Patient: *Yes, but we're a very conservative family when it comes to eating. I can't afford to put food on the table which won't get eaten.*

Practitioner: *Well, perhaps you could start by eating more fruit and veg yourself to set a good example.*

Patient: *Well I know I should do that but...*

Our goal in this book is to take the best of advice-giving, particularly the idea of exchanging information, and place it within a patient-centered framework, with other concepts (readiness, importance and confidence) and more directive practical strategies for guiding quality behavior change discussions. In the face of these refinements, we see little need to hold on to the concept of advice-giving which is so bedeviled by the dangers of direct persuasion. A confrontational interviewing style is too often associated with telling people what to do, and this is likely to lead to resistance (see Chapter 5).

To the reader who finds advice-giving a successful framework for intervention and who remains sceptical about our aversion to direct persuasion we can only say that it is possible that you have found a consulting style based on advice-giving which suits you, and hopefully your patients as well. Much of the content of this book might thus be of cursory interest only. Our suspicion, however, is that if your advice-giving approach works, you are probably doing this with the kind of compassion and quality that is rooted quite firmly in a patient-centered method!

Microskills and strategies

One way of viewing the consultation is to distinguish between microskills, which are used moment-to-moment, and broader strategies which the practitioner uses to guide the direction of the whole process; one moves along two trajectories at the same time. Listening skills are used at the level of microskill on an ongoing basis, to ensure that you understand the patient and that he or she is as active as possible; the strategies, like those described in this book, enable you to be directive.

The patient-centered platform

Patient-centeredness involves more than 'being nice' to patients. It involves careful listening. This is not a passive process, but an active and at times demanding one. In behavior change consultations one might spend time listening carefully to the patient's feeling about readiness, importance and confidence to make a particular change; or one might attend to other, often fundamental, issues like what it feels like to have a particular disease, to come down to the consultation, to have a personal problem, and so on.

Background

A patient- or client-centered method has been constructed in many fields, for example, in psychology, nursing and medicine, where there is no short-age of evidence about the importance of taking into account the patient's perspective when making decisions about treatment and behavior change.

Among the most recent and well-developed statements of the patient-centered method is that provided by Stewart and colleagues (1995):

1. Assessment is when the clinician actively seeks to enter into the patient's world to understand his or her unique experiences of illness. The practitioner explores the patient's ideas about illness, how the patient feels about being ill, what he or she expects from the physician, and how the illness affects the patient's functioning.
2. Ideas about disease (abnormal pathology) and illness (the patient's experience of being unwell) should be integrated with an understanding of the whole person in a broader context.
3. Finding common ground involves both the patient and practitioner working together to define the problem, establish the goals of management and to be clear about the roles expected of doctor and patient.
4. Each contact between clinician and patient should be seen as an opportunity for health promotion.
5. Each contact is an opportunity to develop a therapeutic relationship between clinician and patient.
6. Throughout, the clinician must be realistic about resources (including time and his or her own emotional energy).

Research support for the effectiveness of various elements of the patient-centered method includes demonstration of increased patient satisfaction after seeing the doctor, improved compliance with medication, reduction of patients' concerns, reduction in actual symptoms like raised blood pres-sure, improved postoperative recovery and reduction in blood sugar among people with diabetes (see Orth et al 1987, Kaplan et al 1989, Stewart et al 1995).

The following goals are worth bearing in mind:

- to encourage patients to express concerns
- to help them to be more active in the consultation
- to allow them to articulate what information they require
- to give them greater control of decision making, particularly important when talking about changes in their behavior
- to reach joint decisions.

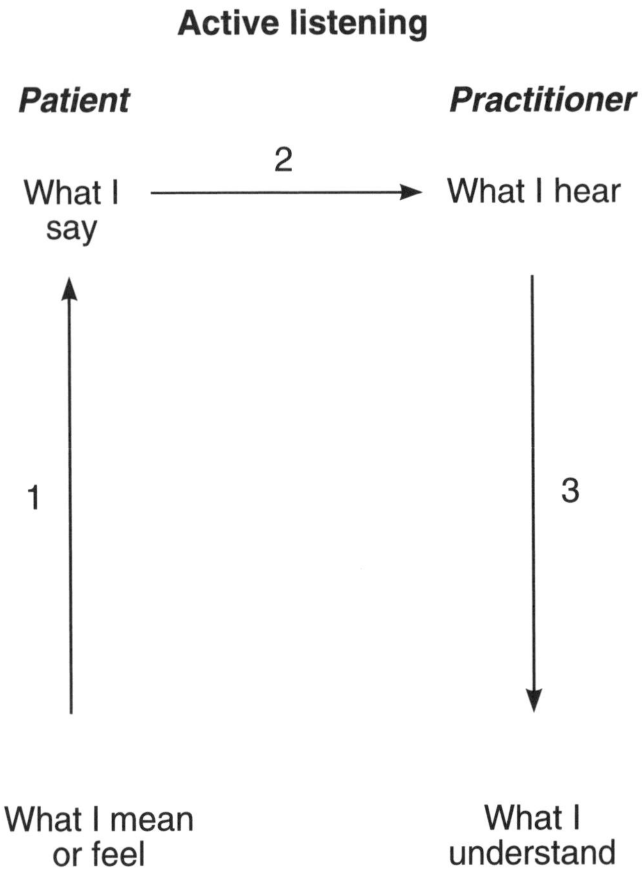

Active listening

| *Patient* | *Practitioner* |

What I
say $\xrightarrow{\quad 2 \quad}$ What I hear

1 ↑   3 ↓

What I mean
or feel

What I
understand

Figure 2.4   Active listening.

Getting it right

To achieve these goals the practitioner needs to encourage, to be curious, to ask open questions and to avoid taking decisions without checking first with the patient. Much more subtle, and critical for the success of this kind of consultation, is to be a good listener, which is not a passive process. Active listening involves searching for an understanding of the underlying meaning beneath the words used by the patient.

This process is illustrated in Figure 2.4, which has been adapted from the work of Thomas Gordon (Gordon 1970, Miller & Jackson 1985). The aim is not to repeat what the patient has said, which is how a computer might carry out this task, but to clarify meaning, a more complex task.

Figure 2.4 illustrates, from bottom left to bottom right, how the meaning being conveyed by the patient can get distorted: first, the patient might not say exactly what she means (see 1). At the second stage, we might not hear what is being said (2). Anyone familiar with strong argument will be familiar with this difficulty. 'I said ...'. 'No you didn't, you said ...'. Mishearing a single word can be sufficient to throw one off course. Third, one might hear the words accurately, but interpret their meaning in quite a different way from the patient (3). Active listening involves bridging the gap between the two meaning boxes.

For example, if a patient says, 'I find it comforting to eat the foods I like', this could be taken to mean a wide range of things by the practitioner. To bridge the gap between the patient's meaning and the practitioner's interpretation involves careful listening, and critically: (1) making a statement designed to clarify meaning (sometimes called reflective listening); or (2) asking a question; or (3) providing a short summary which clarifies the meaning.

Obviously, one needs to do much more than clarify meaning with patients. One might want to encourage decision making, particularly relevant in talk about behavior change. There might be other things on the agenda of the practitioner, which is why we believe that the framework for behavior change consultations should contain more directive elements, to be discussed in the next section. However, if the pursuit of patient concerns and meaning is left behind, communication breakdown will follow, usually in the form of resistance from the patient. Further details about different kinds of reflective listening statements can be found in Miller & Rollnick (1991).

In summary, to achieve the goals of a patient-centered approach, the following techniques should be used:

- Simple open questions.
- Listening and encouraging with verbal and non-verbal prompts.
- Clarifying and summarizing, i.e. checking your understanding of what the patient is saying, or checking the patient's understanding of information given.
- Reflective listening is a higher-level counseling skill which can be extremely useful as well. This involves making statements, the aim of which is to understand the patient's meaning, i.e. to bridge the gap illustrated in Figure 2.4 (see Miller & Rollnick 1991).

To acquire these skills requires practice and self-awareness of what one is doing, and how the patient is responding. Some experienced practitioners say that practice taught them to make simpler contributions to a discussion, not more complex ones. For example, simple open questions like, 'What concerns do you have about your health?' are usually more useful than complex questions like, 'How do you feel about the possibility of losing your good health in the future?' Experienced practitioners say that the less they follow their own agendas and hypotheses, the better they understand their patients.

Negotiation: providing direction in consultations about behavior change

Having described the patient-centered approach, one might stop there and suggest that practitioners can now go forward into behavior change consultations armed with the essential tools of their trade, the patient-centered therapy of 'the word'. Our view is that this might be inadequate, for the following important reason: practitioners and patients often do not feel the same way about behavior change. There is often a tension, a potential for disagreement which one can almost measure like the strength of an electrical current. A patient can resist pressure from a well-meaning practitioner to consider health behavior change. The different agendas of practitioner and patient can play themselves out in a conflict which is sometimes polite, sometimes hidden and repressed, and sometimes open and hostile.

Behavior change consultations have a different quality from those which, for example, focus on breaking bad news to a patient. They are discussions about commitment and resolutions, strategies and obstacles, timing and fine tuning. The subject of change is often raised by the practitioner, and resistance from the patient is much more likely to arise. Moral judgments can be close to the surface of the discussion. Attention is usually focused on what the patient might *do* outside the consulting room. For these reasons, we feel that practitioners need structure to their consultations which provide them with a sense of *direction*, to help them avoid disagreement and achieve congruence. The strategies in Part II of this book are designed to provide this sense of direction.

Practitioners use the term 'directive' in different ways. Because of its association with activities like telling patients what you think they should do, or talking in a forceful way which undermines autonomy, the term often carries a negative connotation. In fact, it is sometimes thought of as representing the very opposite of patient-centeredness! However, this is not what we mean here by providing direction in a consultation.

*The guiding framework for our method is patient-centered **and** directive.* This follows precisely one element of the definition of motivational interviewing (Rollnick & Miller 1995). We use the term 'directive' here to mean *providing structure to a discussion* about behavior change. Within this structure, the best results will be achieved by keeping closely to the principles of patient-centered practice.

It is something of a puzzle to us that no term has emerged to characterize this kind of consultation about behavior change. The term *negotiation* captures the spirit of behavior change consultations fairly well (see Botelho 1992). Here, we are not using the term in a legal or commercial sense, where the artful closing of a deal is sometimes the overriding goal. Rather, it describes the merging of the agendas of practitioner and patient, in which views about behavior change are openly exchanged in a respectful manner. Any good negotiation about behavior change involves careful listening, but also careful guiding (Botelho 1992).

Negotiating behavior change: the spirit of the method

We pay a lot of attention to technique and strategy in this book, yet by far the most important thing is the spirit of the method. Put simply, this is a *collaborative conversation about behavior change.* Rather than wrestling, as a colleague once put it, it is more like dancing (J. Allison, personal communication). The patient is encouraged to be an active decision maker. The practitioner provides structure to the discussion and expert information, where appropriate, and elicits from the patient views and aspirations about behavior change. This is not merely a matter of using techniques or strategies, but of approaching the consultation and the topic of behavior change with a set of attitudes that promote patient autonomy.

Freedom of choice

Most of us behave, at times, in ways that compromise our health, and we each have our own notion of what constitutes 'acceptable risks'. Most of the risks we take are for pleasure or benefit of some kind, or we wouldn't do it!

Our method is based on the principle that, in general, people we meet in consultation usually have the freedom of choice to behave as they wish, within the confines of their social and economic circumstances. Seen in this light, our role is to help them make an informed choice about whether or not to change their behavior. We might want to increase their knowledge of, and access to, healthy options, but their freedom to choose is their fundamental right. If they decide to change, it is our role to help them take effective action based on this choice. It is important to remember that most attempts to change behavior occur naturally, outside of the consultation. We all have experience of this. Sometimes we succeed, and many times we fail.

Since we wish patients to have as much freedom of choice as possible, it is not appropriate to force our views upon them. This method is patient-centered but not without clear direction from the practitioner. The practitioner's role is to help people to make decisions within their own frame of reference. This does not mean that our own views are irrelevant. We do have knowledge about behavior change and about which behaviors are associated with health. However, it is the way in which we share our views with patients that is crucial. An appropriate attitude to behavior change can be described thus: *What do you feel about your — —? How does this fit into your everyday life? I believe that — —, but it is your choice, whether to change or not. If you would like to consider change, remember, I am here to help you if you feel you need this.*

Sometimes, making decisions to change behavior can have profound effects on patients' lives. For example, a simple idea like getting more exercise might seem simple to a practitioner, but in fact can involve a patient in changing a lot in his or her life. Other behaviors might be affected, and the patient might need to examine fears about these changes, for example: *Will taking more exercise lead me to have a heart attack? Will giving up smoking make me put on weight?* Understanding these issues from the patient's point of view might be crucial to your efforts. To achieve this it is necessary to keep close to a basic principle of patient-centered medicine: You must want to understand the patient's perspective. This is both a matter of attitude, and technique. The attitude is one of basic respect. The technical side involves active listening using mostly simple open questions, and reflective listening if you have an interest in this counseling technique.

A few, carefully chosen words, delivered slowly and respectfully, are worth more than many mouthfuls of busy talk. The interviewing style we have found to be particularly useful is a quiet and curious one. This encourages the patient to do most of the talking. Your role is to quietly encourage exploration and decision making. Very simple open questions can be extremely powerful.

It is crucial to respect the autonomy of patients, and their freedom to change or to continue their behavior. Basic counseling skills should be used as a device for understanding, and demonstrating respect for, the patient's views. This is an active, not a passive, process, in which the practitioner tries to empathize with the patient, in other words, see the situation from his or her frame of reference. The patient may come from a different gender/cultural/social background from that of the practitioner, and may have quite different, but equally valid, views and priorities. Conveying respect implies acceptance of whatever decision the patient takes about behavior change.

Your usual consulting style and energy levels

In the course of everyday practice it is not realistic to expect practitioners to use this method in every behaviour change consultation. Sometimes one gets too busy to even raise the subject of behaviour change. Of critical importance is having the stamina to embark on a process of listening and negotiating. Some practitioners, a minority in our experience, are natural listeners, and will not find the use of this method in any way tiring. Others will need to choose the right time to try it out. The most important thing is to make a deliberate decision to change gear, to think about what you are saying to the patient, and to watch his or her response quite carefully.

How do you know when you have got it right?

Some of the key signals are:

- You are speaking slowly.
- The patient is doing much more of the talking than you.
- The patient is actively talking about behavior change.
- You are listening very carefully, and gently directing the interview at appropriate moments.
- The patient appears to be 'working hard', often realizing things for the first time.
- The patient is actively asking for information and advice.
- It feels as if you are holding up a canvas, and the patient is filling it with paint, in places sometimes selected by you, and sometimes by the patient.

Watch your assumptions

Many behavior change consultations fail because the practitioner falls into the trap of making false assumptions. The patient is more likely openly to consider change if you avoid imposing these assumptions on him or her:

1. This person OUGHT to change This is difficult to avoid, because we place a high value on health and often do feel that change would be a good idea. We cannot be dishonest about this. The solution is either to hold back on expressing your views until you understand those of the patient, or to express them openly, but not in an imposing manner, for example: *I think it is a good idea to change your diet, but what do you really think about this?* In other words, express your views in a relatively neutral and non-judgmental way, placing emphasis on the patient's freedom of choice.

2. This person WANTS to change This assumption is easy to avoid. Ask the patient! This is one of the key components of the method, understanding the person's motivation to change. This task is described in detail in Chapter 3. Remember that motivation is not an all-or-nothing phenomenon. It is a question of degree, so do not ask a question like, *Do you or don't you want to reduce your alcohol consumption?* The assessment of how much the person wants to change will be crucial to the success of the consultation. Remember that patients sometimes feel intimidated by health professionals; they might not want to be frank because they fear possible disagreement about behavior change. The practitioner's general attitude and specific wording of questions can help to facilitate honest discussion.

3. This patient's health is the prime motivating factor for him/her This is a very common faulty assumption made in consultations. We become entrapped by our own role as caregivers. For example, fairly healthy patients are not necessarily motivated to change behavior in the interests of long-term health. More immediate prospects like looking better or saving money might be more important. Changing behavior has implications beyond health, and you ignore these at your peril! Not everyone is committed to avoiding bad health.

4. If he or she does not decide to change, the consultation has failed This is unrealistic and too ambitious. Deciding to change is a process, not an event, and it takes time. People vacillate between feeling ready to take action and feeling unwilling to even think about it. Simply helping someone to think a little more deeply about change is a useful outcome of a consultation. A decision to change is more likely to be taken outside of the consultation.

5. Patients are either motivated to change, or not Motivation to do something is not an all-or-nothing phenomenon; it is a matter of degree. Readiness to change varies between individuals, and within them over time.

6. Now is the right time to consider change It might not be! Choosing the right time is a delicate matter. The best guideline is the patient's reactions. If he or she has rushed into the consulting room, late for work after a disagreement at home, you have a problem of timing. Healthcare professionals are used to taking quick decisions in their everyday work. Discussion about a patient's change of lifestyle should not be swamped by this way of dealing with acute medical problems. Choosing the right moment and moving ahead at the right pace will enhance success rates.

7. A tough approach is always best No it is not! Have you ever been encouraged to change by someone who uses this approach? People take a hard line with you when they feel that no other approach is possible. With some patients, on some occasions, being very frank and directly persuasive might be justified and effective, but if you assume this to be necessary for every patient, your efforts will be wasted. Practitioners can enter a vicious circle if they use the tough approach: patients resist (because they do not like feeling cornered), the practitioner feels that they are inherently resistant to change, further tough action appears justified, and so on. A 'Yes, but ...' response from the patient is almost a knee-jerk reaction to being told what to do.

8. I'm the expert. He or she must follow my advice We are not suggesting that your expertise is irrelevant, only that you try to help patients to become more and more expert as well. Telling them what to do is unlikely to achieve this. Also, the way you use your expertise is important. A useful analogy is that of a learner driver who employs a driving instructor. The pupil (or patient) does the driving, and the instructor watches, listens and encourages, making crucial decisions about where to go, how much information to provide, and when to provide it. In consultations about behavior change the patient should be in control. He or she will follow your guidance only for as long as it continues to feel helpful and relevant.

9. A negotiation-based approach is best This is a generalization. A lot more clinical and scientific evidence is needed to justify such a statement. Some patients will respond to a much simpler approach, a kind but firm nudge in what you decide to be the right direction.

Health promotion, values and ethical issues

Ask a group of practitioners if they have the *right* to discourage smoking in their patients and the discussion can get heated. Talk to a heavy-drinking patient about drinking less and you will move rapidly away from medicine into the realms of social custom and personal preference. Some practitioners see no ethical difficulty arising from encouraging patients to change their behavior, even if they have not asked for help. They see it as part of their job to help people to adopt healthier lifestyles. Others argue that encouraging and educating can easily slide into coercing, labeling and blaming. Our view is not to dismiss these concerns, but to identify safeguards for practitioners that encourage good practice and allow for the range of values likely to impinge on talk about behavior change.

Talk about behavior change in the consultation is governed by personal values on both sides. We have deliberately chosen the term 'importance' in this book because it obliges the practitioner to find out what the personal value of change is for each patient. The practitioner's values can be just as powerful a determinant of what is said and done. Without wishing to enter too far into the world of philosophy and linguistics, examination of a statement like 'Smoking is bad for your health and you should consider quitting' can reveal quite a lot more than the apparent discharge of a duty to present evidence of risk to a patient! At its root is a set of values, often keenly felt by practitioners, that revolve around the desirability of controlling one's health and a vision of what a good life is.

Seedhouse (1997) goes so far as to suggest that, for some practitioners, 'it is not objective health concerns which shape their account of the good life, ... it is their understanding of the good life which shapes what they see as health concerns' (p. 96). This issue becomes particularly acute when one is truly in the realm of preventative health promotion, where the patient has no identifiable current health problem. For example, talk to a heavy drinker with no medical problems by following the guidelines for brief intervention laid out in recent research studies, and the potential for value conflict can rise up like a pot of boiling water:

Practitioner: *Have you thought about cutting down your drinking?*

Patient: *I drink the same as all my mates ... I cannot see what the problem is.*

Being aware of how one's values affect practice is a prerequisite for sensitive behavior change discussion.

It can be useful to distinguish between the *goal* of the consultation and the *means* used to achieve that goal. If the clinician's purpose is to encourage behavior change and the patient does not share this goal, ethical difficulties can arise. The obvious safeguard is to be honest with the person about your motives, and to understand his or her point of view. Here, a simple advice-giving approach would seem to be more vulnerable to ethical difficulty than one based on negotiation, because the patient's viewpoint is not necessarily understood.

Assuming some degree of agreement between practitioner and patient about the goal, what about the means used to achieve that end? We do not agree with the assertion that the end justifies the means. Here we find that advice-giving has an apparent simplicity about it: the patient is advised about change and is fully aware of the practitioner's rationale and motives. On the other hand, an approach based on negotiation, using some of the strategies outlined in this book, can sometimes seem less clear to the patient. The practitioner spends quite a lot of time eliciting arguments and solutions from the patient. Where the consultation is going will depend as much on the patient as on the practitioner. Done badly, the practitioner could be seen to be quietly coercive and manipulative.

We suggest that the following safeguards be considered to prevent bad practice. If these are adhered to, we believe that an approach based on negotiation could not only be more effective, but genuinely respectful of the patients.

- Empathy with the patient is paramount. You must want to understand the situation from the patient's point of view.
- Resistance from the patient is a signal to you that rapport is damaged. You can do something about this. It sometimes arises because you are assuming greater readiness to change than is the case, and sometimes because you are asking the patient to examine something which he or she does not want to talk to you about.
- If in any doubt about what you are doing, ask the patient. Be clear and honest.

We would hope that all practitioners are sensitive to ethical dilemmas when dealing with behavior change, and that they are willing to talk to their colleagues (and even their patients) about them. There is no such thing as a purely pragmatic, value-free behavior change consultation!

PRINCIPLES OF GOOD PRACTICE

The above assumptions (pp. 34–36) focus on unproductive attitudes. Put more positively, and by way of summarizing the spirit of behavior change negotiation, the following points capture the essence:

- VALUE BASE
- respect for autonomy of patients and their choices is paramount
- patient should decide what behavior, if any, to focus on (see Chapter 3)
- SKILLS
- a confrontational interviewing style is not productive
- Information exchange is a critical skill (see Chapter 5)
- Readiness to change should be continually monitored (see Chapter 3)
- Importance and confidence should be assessed and responded to (see Chapters 3 and 4)
- ROLES
- *The practitioner*
- Provides structure, direction and support
- Provides information wanted by the patient
- Elicits and respects the patient's views and aspirations
- Negotiates change sensitively
- *The patient*
- Is an active decision maker.

REFERENCES

Ashenden R, Silagy C, Weller D 1997 A systematic review of the effectiveness of promoting lifestyle change in general practice. Family Practice 14:160–175

Botelho R 1992 A negotiation model for the doctor–patient relationship. Family Practice 9:210–218

Davidson R 1998 The transtheoretical model: a critical overview. In: Miller R W, Heather N (eds) Treating addictive behaviors, 2nd edn. Plenum, New York

DiClemente C C, Prochaska J 1998 Toward a comprehensive, transtheoretical model of change: stages of change and addictive behaviors. In: Miller W R, Heather N (eds) Treating addictive behaviors, 2nd edn. Plenum, New York

Gordon T 1970 Parent effectiveness training. Wyden, New York

Grant V J 1995 Therapy of 'the word': new goals in teaching communication skills. Health Care Analysis 3:71–74

Heritage J, Sefi S 1992 Dilemmas of advice: aspects of the delivery and reception of advice in interactions between health visitors and first-time mothers. In: Drew P, Heritage J (eds) Talk at work: interaction in institutional settings. Cambridge University Press, Cambridge

Kaplan S H, Greenfield S, Ware J E 1989 Assessing the effects of physician–patient interactions on the outcomes of chronic disease. Medical Care 27:S110–S127

Miller W R, Heather N (eds) 1998 Treating addictive behaviors, 2nd edn. Plenum, New York

Miller W R, Jackson K A 1985 Practical psychology for pastors: toward more effective counseling. Prentice-Hall, Englewood Cliffs

Miller W R, Rollnick S 1991 Motivational interviewing: preparing people to change addictive behavior. Guilford Press, New York

Orth J E, Stiles W B, Scherwitz L, Hennrikus D, Vallbona C 1987 Patient exposition and provider explanation in routine interviews and hypertensive patients' blood pressure control. Health Psychology 6:29–42

Prochaska J, DiClemente C 1983 Stages and processes of self-change of smoking: towards an integrated model of change. Journal of Consulting and Clinical Psychology 51:390–395

Prochaska J O, DiClemente C C 1986 Towards a comprehensive model of change. In: Miller W R, Heather N (eds) Treating addictive behaviors: processes of change. Plenum, New York

Prochaska J, DiClemente C 1998 Comments, criteria and creating better models: in response to Davidson. In: Miller W R, Heather N (eds) Treating addictive behaviors, 2nd edn. Plenum, New York

Rollnick S 1998 Readiness, importance and confidence: critical conditions of change in treatment. In: Miller W R, Heather N (eds) Treating addictive behaviors, 2nd edn. Plenum, New York

Rollnick S, Miller W R 1995 What is motivational interviewing? Behavioural and Cognitive Psychotherapy 23:325–334

Rollnick S R, Kinnersley P, Stott N 1993 Methods of helping patients with behaviour change. British Medical Journal 307:188–190

Rollnick S, Butler C C, Stott N 1997 Helping smokers make decisions: the enhancement of brief intervention for general medical practice. Patient Education and Counseling 31:191–203

Seedhouse D 1997 Health promotion: philosophy, prejudice and practice. Wiley, Chichester

Silverman D 1997 Discourses in counselling: HIV counselling as social interaction. Sage, London

Stewart M, Stewart M, Belle Brown J et al 1995 Patient-centered medicine: transforming the clinical method. Sage, Thousand Oaks

Stockwell T 1992 Models of change, heavenly bodies and weltanschuungs. British Journal of Addiction 87:830–831

PART II

The tasks

Getting started: rapport, agendas and assessment

This chapter describes the early tasks in negotiating behavior change. These are to establish rapport, to set the agenda and to assess importance and confidence about changing a specific behavior. (See Figure 3.1.)

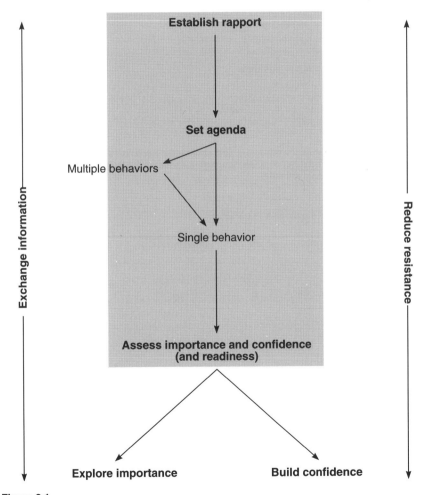

Figure 3.1

Box 3.1 Useful Questions

Establish rapport
Any question that you think might help you understand the patient better will be useful. If time is available consider using the 'Typical Day' strategy (see p. 112).

Set agenda

Multiple behaviors

1. *What would you like to talk about today? We could talk about smoking, exercise, eating or drinking all of which affect your recovery from the heart attack. But what do you think? Perhaps you are more concerned about something else?*
2. *Would you like to talk about any changes to your health like eating or smoking, or have you come here today with other concerns on your mind?*
3. *Which of exercise or diet do you feel most ready to talk about?*

Single behaviors

1. *Some people find that changing x* [behavior] *can improve y* [condition]. *What do you think?*
2. *I am concerned about your chest. I wonder how you feel about your smoking?*
3. *How does your use of alcohol affect this problem* [the presenting complaint]?

Assess importance and confidence

Assess importance
How do you feel at the moment about [change]? *How important is it to you personally to –* [change]? *If 0 was 'not at all important' and 10 was 'very important', what number would you give yourself?*

Assess confidence
If you decided right now to – [change], *how confident do you feel about succeeding with this? If 0 stands for 'not at all confident' and 10 stands for 'very confident', what number would you give yourself?*

TASK: ESTABLISH RAPPORT

Practitioner: *Your blood pressure is a bit higher than when I last saw you.*

Patient: *Really?*

Practitioner: *Yes, do you remember about how best to control it?*

Patient: *Well, I do take my tablets.*

Practitioner: *All of the time, or do you miss them out sometimes?*

Patient: *No, its fine. I take them.* [Silence]

Practitioner: *What about your diet?*

Patient: *That's fine too. I mean I don't eat too much. Like everyone else, I have my lapses, but I'm OK.*

Sometimes it is difficult to get started on a discussion about behavior change. Good rapport is essential for an honest discussion and for constructive understanding of patients' behavior and openness to change. It is not always necessary to labor this task. Rapport is sometimes quickly established or re-established, and the agenda is often obvious. In some settings, for example in primary healthcare, there may already be an existing relationship between health professional and patient and this will provide a backdrop to the current consultation. In other settings, for example a first appointment with a dietitian, a relationship will need to be established quickly. Rapport is easy to understand and recognize, although sometimes it is taken for granted. It can be difficult to repair once damaged.

How not to do it!

Ignore this step altogether and launch straight into whatever you consider to be the agenda for the consultation. Ideally avoid eye contact and use of the patient's name while doing this!

> Practitioner: [looking at notes as patient enters] *So, have you given up smoking yet?*

Towards good practice

It is not difficult to get things off to a good start. The guidelines below are basic but essential for avoiding damage to rapport. Premature focus, a topic to be discussed in the next section of this chapter, is the most common cause for this damage.

Physical setting

The physical setting for the consultation may either promote or obstruct the development of the rapport. An equal power relationship is essential for successful negotiation. Consider the following factors which may affect this:

- Is the patient's first encounter in the clinic one in which he or she will be listened to, even if for just a few minutes? Or is he or she obliged to undergo routine testing which is primarily of concern to the practitioner?
- Privacy for the patient.
- Shared access to notes.
- Appropriate wall posters.
- The practitioner's style of dress: does it unnecessarily suggest a power imbalance?
- Has everyone in the room (e.g. students) been introduced?

Thoughts and feelings about the consultation

The patient's expectations will affect rapport. He or she will expect or hope to be handled by the practitioner in a certain way. Check these and clarify any misunderstandings. The patient may also have come with immediate problems or concerns which will need addressing before he or she will be comfortable about addressing other matters like behavior change. It is important to identify these and respond appropriately.

It is also worth acknowledging the context of the consultation for the patient, and his or her feelings about this, for example: *I'm sorry you've been kept waiting – at the end of the day I expect you're impatient to get home.* or *It must have been a worrying time for you since your heart attack* [diabetes diagnosis, etc.] *and I know you've already seen several other members of the team to discuss ways to keep you healthy in the future.*

It may be necessary to switch focus from *treating* the patient to *negotiating* behavior change. After giving an injection, doing a dressing or some other procedure where the patient has (appropriately) been a more or less passive recipient of your ministrations, there will need to be a clear change in focus: *Now that's out of the way let's sit down and think together about some of the other things affecting your* —'.

If the patient feels respected and cared for from the beginning, any subsequent discussion will be easier.

Additional strategy: a typical day

One useful strategy for establishing rapport is to use a strategy called 'A Typical Day', which is described in detail in Chapter 5, where its benefit to information exchange is highlighted (see p. 112). Here the patient describes a typical day, and usually says where the behavior under discussion fits into this context. The practitioner's role is to practise restraint and develop an interest in the layers of personal detail provided. It is also useful close to the beginning of a consultation, even if the subject of behavior change has not been raised. If one has time to spare, say 6–8 minutes, it can be a most worthwhile experience for both parties. One can follow the account of a typical day in general, without reference to any behavior. If carried out skillfully, rapport will be strengthened immeasurably.

TASK: SET AGENDA

Jennifer, 35 years old and asthmatic, finds it very difficult to remember to take her medication regularly, smokes 20 cigarettes a day, works in a bar in a very smoky atmosphere and is very inactive. She says that after being on her feet all night the last thing she wants to do in her spare time is exercise!

Sometimes there are so many things contributing to a person's poor health that it is hard to know where to begin.

Of all the judgments made in a behavior change consultation the poorest often arise from a premature leap into specific discussion of a change, when the patient is more concerned about something else. Indeed, this kind of premature leap can become almost institutionalized in a treatment setting, where patients are encouraged to change their behavior before they are ready for it (see Chapter 8, p. 194).

Sometimes it can be a relatively mundane matter which prevents a focus on behavior change: a patient who arrives at a consultation upset about a minor car accident might not be able to concentrate well on anything the practitioner says. Sometimes it is a personal matter that the patient is more concerned with, and *might* want to talk about; someone who has recently had a heart attack might be preoccupied with matters of life and death. To talk about getting more exercise under these circumstances could be poorly timed, even insensitive. A critical early task therefore is to *agree the agenda*.

Even when behavior change *is* a viable topic for discussion, one is often faced with multiple, interrelated health behaviors. For example, many excessive drinkers also smoke. Thus, health behaviors deemed to be risky often coexist in individuals. Sufferers from diabetes, heart disease and other chronic conditions frequently face the challenge of changing more than one behavior. Deciding what to talk about is thus a crucial first step.

We have made a distinction in this chapter between single and multiple behavior change discussions when setting an agenda. We advise practitioners to make a clear and conscious choice between using either Strategy 1 or 2 (for multiple behaviors) or Strategy 3 (for a single behavior). This is because we have noticed so many practitioners who, when faced with a range of possible behaviors, prematurely oblige a patient to discuss one particular behavior at the expense of others. If someone is more ready to change their pattern of exercise than their diet, why focus on diet? *At this stage of the consultation our assumption is that the patient should be given control of its direction.*

The guidelines for Strategy 1, *agenda setting*, are based on the use of an agenda-setting chart. This was originally developed in a general health promotion setting (Rollnick & Mason 1992), and then refined and adapted by a team working on a negotiating method for use among sufferers from Type II diabetes (see Stott et al 1995). Practitioners (nurses and doctors) were trained in a flexible way, according to their interest in receiving input from a trainer who visited their practices over a period of 3 years. Initial training took the form of a brief 1-hour session, approximately half of which focused on the use of the agenda-setting procedure. Two findings of particular interest emerged from the follow-up of practitioners (Stott et al 1996): first, nurses seemed more receptive, on the whole, than doctors, although evidence of inventiveness and adaptability was also apparent within the latter group. Second, over 80% of practitioners reported using the chart in consultations with other patients, sometimes with other behavior change difficulties. It is therefore a relatively simple procedure to teach and use, although documented evidence of its validity is thus far confined to the above study in the diabetes field.

The guidelines for Strategy 2, *talking about stress*, are based on the use of a *stress bucket* which emerged from experimentation in stress management groups in a primary healthcare setting. It has not been formally evaluated, but we know that it has face validity with patients, as a device for structuring a discussion about stress and making a decision about what to do next. It has been used with both individuals and groups.

STRATEGY 1: MULTIPLE BEHAVIORS – AGENDA SETTING

Negotiating behavior change is a specific process. It is applicable to a range of behaviors but can only be used with regard to one specific behavior at a time. It is not possible effectively to negotiate a 'healthier lifestyle in general'. We are all at different stages of readiness to change over different issues. Even within one topic such as diet we may be ready to make one change (e.g. eat more fruit) but not ready to make another (e.g. eat less fat). Sometimes changing one behavior will have a knock-on effect on another but it is important to keep the process to one behavior at a time. When there is a range of behaviors that could be discussed it is essential to prioritize and focus upon one clear objective. This makes the whole process more manageable. How do you decide what to talk about?

How not to do it!

Make your own decision about what your patients' priorities should be, tell them so, and proceed accordingly. Ideally, go through each behavior in turn, and make sure that you identify change targets for each one. Use a checklist approach, so common in everyday medicine.

> So, let's start with deciding what you are going to do about giving up smoking. When we've agreed a quit date and fixed you up with a support group to attend we can go on to look at this business of forgetting to take your inhalers. Having sorted out those urgent issues we can consider how you can get away from all the passive smoking at work and get some exercise a couple of times a week. Okay?

Towards good practice

The aim here is to be open and honest about your agenda, to understand the patient's agenda, and to help the patient select a behavior, if appropriate. The patient might, however, prefer to talk about a pressing personal matter. The practitioner's behavior and tone of voice should reflect an attitude of curiosity about what the patient really wants to talk about. This agenda setting can be done informally by asking a series of *open questions*. Here are some examples:

> *Before we get down to any details, what would you like to talk about? Changing your diet, getting more exercise, or is there something else that's more pressing for you today?*

> *What would you like to talk about today? We could talk about smoking, exercise, eating or drinking, all of which affect your recovery from the heart attack. But what do you think? Perhaps you are more concerned about something else?*

> *Can we just stand back a moment? Tell me how you would like to spend this time together? I usually talk to people in a situation like yours about smoking, food, exercise, tablets, and that sort of thing. How do you feel, which of these do you feel most ready to change, or is there something else bothering you?*

We have found that the use of an *agenda-setting chart* (Fig. 3.2) is one way of doing this. It not only saves time, but involves you in a collaborative exercise which maximizes patient choice. Remember that this chart is merely an aid to dialog. The technology should not get in the way. It can be just

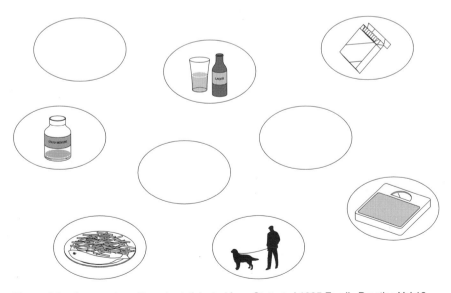

Figure 3.2   An agenda-setting chart. Adapted from Stott et al 1995 Family Practice Vol 12 No 4 pp 413–416 Fig 1, Oxford University Press, with permission of the publisher.

as useful to conduct this negotiation without any technology, by simply asking a set of open questions.

The agenda-setting chart shown in Figure 3.2 illustrates a range of health behaviors. The chart has blank spaces on it to represent issues or behaviors which the patient feels might affect the possibility of behavior change, for example, a spouse who smokes, financial worries which affect the purchase of different food, or a more pressing personal problem such as feeling depressed. Using the chart also allows the practitioner to openly acknowledge what behaviors he or she is concerned about. The aim is to encourage the patient to decide what to talk about, assisted by the practitioner.

- It can be helpful to write on the chart, or even to ask the patient to do this. For example, in the blank spaces you can fill in a concern raised by the patient. You might put a cross through a behavior that is not relevant (e.g. 'I don't smoke'). Or you might even write a specific target underneath a circle, and suggest that the patient takes the chart home.
- Exchanging information can be a crucial part of this review (see Chapter 5).
- The two most common dangers when using this chart are a tendency to use it as a checklist and being in a hurry, which usually leads to a premature focus on one behavior at the expense of others.
- The chart should not be given to practitioners without prior training in its use.

Introduce the agenda-setting chart

For example: *On this card there is a range of things which can affect people's health. Those which most affect* [patient's condition, if appropriate] *are* ——. *How do you feel about these? Are you ready to think about changing any of them? These blank spaces are for any other things which you think might be of greater concern to you today. What do you think? What would you like to talk about today?*

Note that there is a difference between saying to the patient, 'Are you ready **to think about** changing any of …?' (used above), and saying, 'Are you ready to change any of …?'. More patients will be responsive to the former approach than the latter, which implies a greater degree of readiness to change.

Another example: *On this card here are some of the things which affect people's health. I wonder whether you might be interested in talking about changing your diet or smoking, but what do you think? You will be the best judge of what to consider changing. Are there any that you think we could talk about? Or do you have other concerns today* [pointing to blank circles] *which are more pressing?*

Deal with other concerns

Practitioners often say that the blank circles are the most useful part of the agenda-setting chart. If patients identify some other issue or concern, be careful not to assume that they want to talk about it. Someone might say that his car has just broken down and he wants to get home as soon as possible.

However, if the patient does want to talk about something, the challenge is to listen and advise (if advice is wanted), and then decide where to go next, all in a brief period of time. Do not assume that because patients want to talk about an issue, they want a psychotherapy session! We have found that they are usually aware of time constraints, and that a few minutes of careful listening is much appreciated. At a certain point you, and hopefully the patient as well, will be happy to 'park' this discussion. At that point, you might say something like: *We have talked about — —, and I can understand why this must be bothering you. Where does this leave us now? Would you be happy to move on to talk about other things?* It can be useful to write this concern into one of the blank spaces on the agenda-setting chart.

Discuss the range of behaviors

Take care not to push the patient into a premature focus on any one behavior. Listen and elicit. Get yourself into a curious state of mind. You really want to know exactly how the person feels about the selection of a topic to talk about.

You can use the *readiness rule* (see p. 69) to help with this task. Your goal is to find out which behavior the patient is most ready to talk about. For example:

Which of these do you feel most ready to think about changing?

What exactly are you saying about your smoking and drinking? How ready do you feel to talk about changing them, or would you prefer to leave it for the time being?

Thinking about getting more exercise, where would you place yourself on this line? Some people are not at all ready, some are very ready, and others are somewhere in between. How do you feel about this at the moment?

Summarize the outcome

Summarize your understanding of the outcome, and be prepared for any of these possibilities:

- The patient is not interested in changing any behavior, in which case your discussion could end here.
- The patient is willing to talk about changing a specific behavior.
- The patient is ambivalent about a particular behavior.

Consider a more detailed examination of the importance of change, and the building of confidence (Chapter 4). If time is running out, you might consider asking the patient to keep a diary of the behavior, or simply to go away and think about it.

A note about patient autonomy   The emphasis on patient autonomy in this stage of the consultation, and indeed in all of the strategies described in this book, can be misunderstood by practitioners. It can be used as a vehicle for reinforcing pessimism and even a form of passive aggression, borne of frustration from dealing with particularly difficult behavior change encounters. *It's not up to me, it's up to the patient. If he wants to die young, that's his problem.* We have encountered practitioners using the agenda-setting strategy described below with this kind of attitude towards the process. Besides the obvious need to take stock of one's own feelings about the lack of patient progress in one's work, it can be useful to remember that we are not talking here about being guided by a simple notion of directiveness versus non-directiveness. The practitioner is very directive in using the agenda-setting strategy described above, in defining the task and seeing it through to a satisfactory outcome. At the same time he or she is also patient-centered, in encouraging the patient to take control of a topic for discussion. It is a vehicle for genuine negotiation, for having a sensitive and purposeful conversation about change.

A note about checklists   The worst way to use the agenda-setting chart is as if it is a checklist, controlled by the practitioner, in which the patient is asked to go through each behavior in turn. This loses the spirit of the task. This strategy should therefore *not* be used without adequate training in its use.

A note about feeling blamed   We have found that the agenda-setting process is sometimes clouded by an issue which prevents it from being used constructively: the focus on changing lifestyle and encouraging the patient to take responsibility leads the patient to feel blamed for having the problem in the first place, or at least blamed for not ensuring that progress is made. Observation that the patient is not engaged in agenda setting can be a clue that this problem is emerging. The patient's feelings about this need to be understood before continuing with the agenda-setting process.

A note about the use of visual aids   Remember that visual aids like the agenda-setting chart are just that, and no more. If it does not feel comfortable to use it, don't! It is the general spirit of the encounter that is important.

STRATEGY 2: MULTIPLE BEHAVIORS – TALKING ABOUT STRESS

We might argue about how to define stress, but many patients see this as a central force in their lives.

A lorry driver has a heart attack

Practitioner: *It's good to see that you are feeling so much better. I see that you are going home in a few days?*

Patient: *Yes, I don't know, it's a frightening thought, there's too much going on out there and I don't know where to start.*

Practitioner: *What concerns you the most?*

Patient: *Well, you people say that I must stay off work for at least a month but then it will be madness at work; my boss will have no sympathy at all, he just wants me back on the road in that truck today.*

Practitioner: *As if you've just been on holiday or something.*

Patient: *Exactly.*

Practitioner: *Do you know about what is going to help with your recovery in the way of changes in your lifestyle?*

Patient: *Well, you people have given me all the lectures, as if it's really simple, 'just get more exercise, watch your diet, drink less'. If I stop smoking I get crazy and restless, so now you want me to get even more stressed than I already am. And now I have the biggest problem of them all: when am I going to drop dead from another heart attack?*

The sense of being overwhelmed by pressures and problems is not something confined to executives, to be read about in airport lounges, but is pervasive across all strata of western society. One of us recently came across a mother living alone with seven children, without support from family or friends. Like the lorry driver described above, she simply did not know where to begin to feel better and more in control.

Many behavior change discussions have stress as an underlying theme. Rather than leave this topic to one side, it can be helpful to bring it out into the open, and consider what behavior changes, if any, might help. The *stress bucket* is simply a device for structuring this discussion. It has been adapted from a model of stress described by Powell & Enright (1990). The way in which it is used is critical. The goal is to provide a clear structure, and within this to encourage the patient to think and talk about changes. It is a different way of setting an agenda.

A note about inappropriate use This strategy should never be used as standard practice in an insensitive way. On a few occasions, with people who are feeling particularly helpless, we have found that the strategy merely leads to the conclusion that there is nothing the patient can do. Very little constructive discussion emerges. If you are genuinely trying to understand how someone feels, then such a conclusion does not harm the person, because he or she at least feels understood.

How not to do it

Identify stress as a problem, and tell the patient what you think he or she should do about it: *It's quite obvious that you are under stress at the moment. I suggest that you take things one at a time, and begin with your diet. Cut back on fatty foods, and let's get your weight down to begin with. Then we can talk about other things, OK?* The patient will respond with *Mhmm*, and you can be fairly sure that you have missed the mark.

Towards good practice

The aim here is to use the stress bucket (Fig. 3.3) to help the person to take an initially very broad view of stress, its causes and consequences. Having done this, if you sit back and are prepared to tolerate a period of uncertainty with the patient, he or she will often lead you to talk about a change. The strategy follows a similar pattern to the *elicit–provide–elicit* sequence for information exchange (see p. 111). A genuinely curious tone needs to be adopted in the first and third phases, where the practitioner sits back and tries to understand how the patient sees things.

ELICIT personal views and feelings about stress

- Elicit permission to talk about stress.
- Encourage the patient to tell you about why he or she is under stress (causes) or how it is affecting them (symptoms).

Why are you under stress at the moment?

What sort of things make you feel under stress?

How does it affect you?

How does it affect your body/moods/everyday life?

PROVIDE explanation: introduce bucket

- Emphasize that stress is normal.
- Explain how causes, symptoms and solutions are represented on the diagram. Do not feel the need to personalize matters now; leave that for

Your stress levels

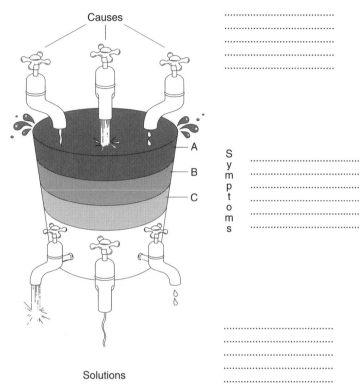

Figure 3.3 A stress bucket. Adapted from Powell & Enright 1990 Anxiety and Stress Management, Routledge, London, Figs 4.2 & 4.3, with permission of the publisher.

later, once the patient has understood the diagram. For example, it might be introduced thus, referring to other people rather than to the patient.

Everyone has some amount of stress in their lives. In fact, without some amount of stress in the bucket, you would never get out of bed in the morning! But why does the level of stress rise in the bucket? Well, everyone has different causes or reasons why the bucket gets filled up. These are the causes up here [point to taps]. *They fill the bucket …* [and continue].

- *Causes* are the things that *fill the bucket* (see taps). Some can be changed others not. Some come in a torrent, others in a steady, though small, drip-drip form.
- *Symptoms* are the things that happen to you *as the level rises*. They affect the body (e.g. heart rate, aches and pains, dizziness), the mind (e.g. poor concentration and memory, feeling tired, worrying too much) and behaviour (e.g. difficulty with sleep, smoking / drinking / eating habits).

- *Solutions* are the things that *lower the level in the bucket* (taps beneath bucket) (e.g. talking to someone about worries, relaxation, exercise, altering one of the causes).

ELICIT personal reactions (causes/symptoms/solutions)

Here the practitioner sits back and allows the patient to set the agenda, using simple questions like:

What do you make of that?

What about your situation?

Can you see how you would fill this in for your situation?

You can focus the discussion on one section of the bucket using questions like:

What happens to you as the level rises? (symptoms)

What's filling your bucket at the moment? (causes)

What helps you to release stress? (solutions)

TALK about change

The discussion often leads to talk about change. If this happens, be careful not to close this down prematurely. Patients can sometimes seem confused and silences can follow as they talk about the possibilities. The only guideline is to stay with them and retain a genuinely curious tone which reflects the underlying spirit of the exercise:

You are the best judge of what will work for you. It's not essential to make decisions now. Our aim is just to have a look at the situation.

If a particular change is identified, then one can use any of the strategies outlined in the following pages and chapters. Some patients are happy to take away an incomplete drawing of the bucket, to fill this in at a later time. Others choose to return for further discussion if this is made available.

STRATEGY 3: SINGLE BEHAVIOR – RAISE SUBJECT

In some circumstances the health professional has clearly identified one particular behavior which he or she wants to discuss. Where the setting is a particular clinic, for example a stop-smoking group, the agenda is clear and explicit to both patient and health professional: there is no need to worry about how best to raise the issue. Other situations are less straightforward and are most often in the context of a patient presenting with a particular symptom or disorder and the health professional identifying a probable or certain link with a particular behavior. Alternatively, as a result of a health check it may be that there is a single behavior that is clearly compromising the patient's best health.

Some practitioners do not believe that this is a particularly sensitive matter. They believe that it is their professional duty to raise a concern about risky health behavior and that not raising the issue would be to shirk this responsibility. We do not accept this as an overriding assumption. We have seen too many patients shifting uncomfortably in their seats when a problem raised by the practitioner 'hits them in the face'. Also, we are aware of some research findings where interviews with patients suggest that they have strong views about it (see Stott & Pill 1990). Of critical importance is the quality of rapport between the parties.

How not to do it!

Raise the subject in an abrupt, patronizing and judgmental way, without having established any rapport with the patient beforehand. *I think we both know you've been a bit naughty about your* [drinking, diet, etc.], *don't we?* or *I think you've brought this on yourself by smoking, haven't you?* Direct confrontation will in most cases elicit resistance. Be ready for the *Yes, but …* response.

Towards good practice

If you have good rapport with someone, you can talk about any subject. Therefore, consider this your first priority. Remember that you and the patient are both on the same side: you both have an interest in improving or maintaining his or her health. Be honest about your own agenda and invite the patient to express his or her own views on the subject. For example:

I've been wondering what is the most important thing we should concentrate on to improve your health at the moment. I think it would help a lot if you could lose some of that excess weight. How does it seem to you? What do you think the priority should be?

[This condition] is sometimes linked with, or caused by [behavior]. I wonder if we could talk briefly about whether that might apply to you?

Have you ever considered whether getting more exercise might improve control of the diabetes?

How do you feel about the amount you drink?

Did you know that some people find that changing [behavior] can help improve [condition]?

*I'm concerned about your chest. I wonder how **you** feel about your smoking.*

People who do [behavior] *are at greater risk of developing* [condition]. *Would you be interested in talking through whether it might be worth your while to change?*

Be clear that your interest in the behavior is not because you think the patient should not be doing it but because you think there may be some health benefits for them in changing. Because of this your inquiry and concern are legitimate and non-judgmental. At this stage the subject is raised for discussion only, with the question of change still open.

The delicate subject

There are some occasions when raising the subject can be undoubtedly difficult. There is no easy formula here, other than by taking time to establish good rapport. Raising the subject of heavy drinking is a good example. A proud person who feels concerned about being stigmatized as an alcoholic can make things difficult for the clinician concerned about his or her health. The mere mention of the word 'alcohol' produces immediate resistance. Put bluntly, as a Norwegian colleague has observed, undermine someone's self-esteem and he or she will resist your efforts (Tom Barth, personal communication). Under these circumstances, it seems easier to say what one should not do. Obviously, no reference should be made to words like 'alcoholic', 'problem', or even 'concern'. Leave it up to the patient to reach this kind of conclusion. *Use of alcohol* is the safest phrase to use. If one encounters immediate resistance, this is a signal to change strategy.

In truth, we have not found an easy route through this problem; no simple strategy that will unlock a patient's willingness to talk, apart from conveying a genuine concern for the person. For example, one of us came across a 45-year-old male patient who simply stopped eating in the face of enormous pressure at home. He had three children under the age of five years, one of whom had a serious respiratory problem. His partner was suffering from post-natal depression and dependence on alcohol. He was seriously sleep deprived and under stress at work. Eventually he was admitted to hospital, passing blood in his urine. Through a series of complicated investigations, which included exploratory surgery, he remained passive and silent. One day, out of the blue, his anaesthetist came to his bedside, closed the door, sat beside him, and asked what he thought might have caused his symptoms. The floodgates opened, and the patient acknowledged his problems at home. He was discharged from hospital soon afterwards, into the care of a psychologist. He said that this anaesthetist was the only person who had seemed genuinely concerned about him as a person.

A productive way of building this kind of rapport is to use the Typical Day strategy (see p. 112). This immediately places a subject like alcohol use or unhealthy eating behavior in a normal context, and protects you from becoming too investigative or confrontational (e.g. *How much do you really drink?*). You might introduce the strategy like this:

> *I really do not know a lot about you and the kind of life you lead. Perhaps we can spend a few minutes with you telling me about a typical day in your life, from beginning to end. If you like, as you go along, you can tell me where your diet, use of alcohol and exercise fit in.*

If you raise the subject and get the impression that the person is feeling threatened, it can be useful to give him or her time to think. This is fairly easy in a primary healthcare setting, where continuity of care is a possibility. The person can come back and see you again. Back off in a non-threatening way, and come back to it later. Even in a hospital setting, we have found it useful to leave the person's bedside for a while and come back to the discussion at a later point in time. If a patient knows that your concern is genuine, and you have a reasonable rapport between you, the boredom of hospital routine can make your return visit more interesting to the patient than you might expect.

TASK: ASSESS IMPORTANCE, CONFIDENCE AND READINESS

> *I'd love to give up smoking. I know it's bad for my health, the kids hate me smoking and it is becoming even more of a problem now that my workplace has become a no-smoking area. I just don't seem to be able to though. I've tried half a dozen times and the longest I last is about 3 weeks so I've just about given up trying.*

> *I could cut down my drinking any time if I really wanted to. When I went on that diet 2 years ago I didn't drink at all for 6 weeks. But I don't see any need to cut down at the moment. I'm fit, I never get bad hangovers and it doesn't interfere with my work or my family. If I saw the need I would just get on and do it.*

It seems that some people cannot change and others do not want to.

Having agreed to talk about a particular behavior there are a number of directions one could take. We have found that the assessment of importance and confidence is a useful first step, hence our decision to use this as the fulcrum for decision making in this method. Put simply, it helps you understand exactly what someone feels about change. We are not suggesting that this task should be carried out in *every* consultation. One might, for example, know how a patient feels about change, or at least have a strong intuition about this. You might decide to carry out another task, for example exchanging information (Chapter 5), or use a strategy for exploring importance (see Chapter 4). If the consultation is like a journey, assessing importance and confidence is one route that could be taken.

We have suggested that a person's readiness to change (a more global concept) is influenced by his or her perceptions of importance and confidence, i.e. he or she should explain his or her stated position on a readiness to change continuum (see Chapter 2, Fig. 2.2, p. 20) Someone might be convinced of the *personal value* of change (*importance*) but not feel confident about mastering the skills necessary to achieve it (*confidence*). This applies to many smokers. Heavy drinkers, on the other hand, can be quite different: they often have mixed feelings about the value of change (*importance*) but say that they could achieve this fairly easily (*confidence*) if they really wanted to. When it comes to changes in eating patterns, people often have relatively low levels on both dimensions.

One can assess readiness in addition to importance and confidence (see Strategy 2 below). Particular emphasis, however, will be placed on importance and confidence, given the subtle interaction between them in everyday practice.

The assessment can be done informally by simply asking the patient to clarify how he or she feels about importance and confidence. It can also be done more formally, using a standard set of questions, something we have found particularly useful in training exercises (see de Shazer et al 1986). In either case the assessment can take as little as 2–3 minutes.

The more standardized assessment procedure emerged from experimentation with smokers (Rollnick et al 1997, Butler et al, in press). Our starting point was a need to develop a method that we could teach to family practitioners for use in consultations lasting 7–10 minutes. Our goal was to find a way of conducting a quick psychological assessment of smoking, i.e. 2–3 minutes, which could lay the foundation for a conversation about change. In our pilot work with a group of volunteer smokers, we began with a readiness to change continuum, hoping to use this as a guide to the choice of strategy the practitioner might use. Initially we became confused by the fact that people placing themselves in similar positions on a readiness continuum had such different needs. The choice of strategy was not immediately apparent from the person's stated readiness to change. We started asking them *why* they had put a mark on a given point on the continuum, and then it struck us that the conversations tended to embrace two topics, importance and confidence, as we described in Chapter 2 (see p. 20). We then decided to assess these dimensions directly, and developed a single-page intervention method, based on this assessment, which was used for training practitioners (Rollnick et al 1997). We also found that they subsequently used this assessment in everyday practice, and not just with smokers, but in other behavior change discussions. When used in our own consultations, with other kinds of behavior change problems, very few patients have difficulty with the numerical scaling technique on which the assessment is based. Of course, this depends crucially on the specificity and relevance of the change under discussion. The more specific the change, the easier is it to understand the assessment.

In essence, this assessment of importance and confidence is a structured and directive way of enabling patients to say how they feel about a particular change within a couple of minutes. Its orientation is patient-centered: it provides a platform for responding to the domain defined by the patient as most in need of attention. The choice of strategy within each domain is dealt with in the following chapter. Our focus here is merely on assessment.

STRATEGY 1: ASSESS IMPORTANCE AND CONFIDENCE

How not to do it

Skip this task altogether. Assume that you know whether you should focus on perceived importance or confidence. You could also assume that the building of confidence is your priority, because it is easier to talk about concrete targets than more subtle matters like the personal value of change to the individual. If resistance arises, blame the patient!

> *So, we both know how important it is for you to lose weight. Let's find a diet that you think would work for you and book you into our slimmers' club to give you some moral support. I can see you don't look very enthusiastic, but you're really going to have to commit yourself to this, this time, if it's going to work.*

Towards good practice

The assessment can be done *informally*. The following example illustrates the informal process of unraveling which dimension is of greatest concern to the patient, in this case, in a conversation about exercise.

Informal assessment of importance and confidence

> Practitioner: *So, we have identified that you get very little exercise since you were promoted to an office-based job, and consequently you have put on some weight. You also find the new job stressful and could do with a way of letting off steam. How do you feel about organizing some sort of physical activity for yourself now you are not in a physically demanding job?*

> Patient: *Well, I can see the need. I don't like feeling so unfit and I've never had such a belly on me in my life! I can't see myself paying out good money to go to a gym just to pump iron for the sake of it though. When I was loading lorries and so on there was a purpose to it. I never stick with things I don't think are useful.*

Practitioner: *So you like being active if you're achieving something that's important to you. Have you ever been into sport? Ball games?*

Patient: *Not really. Although I used to be strong I was never much good at the skill side and games are not much fun if you're no good at them. It's hard to think what I could do that would, like you say, help me to let off steam and keep me in trim. I'd like to find something though.*

It quickly becomes clear that the patient understands and believes in the importance of change but will need some help to think creatively about how to go about it. He has no confidence that he would be able to pursue the solutions he can see at present.

We have found that it is useful to adopt a curious manner during this process, since this reflects your genuine confusion about how the patient really feels. It is not a question–answer session that you are completely in control of, but rather a matter of asking the patient to paint a picture: you are sitting back and allowing the patient to do most of the talking, leaving silences if necessary.

When doing a more formal assessment, the patient must be actively involved. You provide the structure, and the patient does the rest. If it looks or feels like a question–answer assessment session, then you are falling short of the ideal.

- The assessment can be done verbally, or by using lines drawn on a piece of paper. If you use paper, it can be less confusing to use separate sheets.
- The spirit of this exercise is most important. You need to feel genuinely *curious*. It is not an investigation, but an inquiry.
- The goal of the assessment is to work out which of the two domains, importance or confidence, should be focused on.
- The words one uses can be critical: for example, a smoker talking about quitting might respond differently to questions about her confidence to 'have a go', 'stop for a week' or 'never touch a cigarette again'.

Introduce the assessment

The patient should fully understand why you would like to use this strategy, and rapport should be good. Its introduction can be delivered thus:

*I am not really sure **exactly** how you feel about* [behavior or change]. *Can you help me by answering two simple questions, and then we can see where to go from there?*

[Pause, and deal with whatever response patients make. Sometimes they do not allow you to get going, and proceed to tell you how they feel! This is exactly what you want. Leave the assessment aside, and return to it if you are still confused.]

If the patient seems disengaged, then do not do the assessment. Attempt to raise the level of engagement first. Express curiosity. If your rapport is good enough, you can challenge the patient in a friendly way, for example:

> *Have you ever sat down with someone and said exactly how you feel about* [behavior or change]?

Or you can deliberately make the avoidance of premature focus explicit:

> *In a discussion like this it can be a mistake to jump too quickly to talk about doing this or doing that. I certainly don't want you to feel pressurized in any way. We could talk about something else?*

Assess importance

There is no one way of doing this, and we certainly do not have enough experience of different situations to be dogmatic about this. The most direct question would be something like this:

> *How do you feel **at the moment** about* [change]? *How **important** is it to you personally to* [change]? *If 0 was 'not important' and 10 was 'very important', what number would you give yourself?*

Sometimes a patient will simply respond by saying 'very important'. In this case, you can move directly into the process of exploring importance described in the next chapter. A useful and obvious response is simply to ask, 'Why?'. The answer will amount to a series of self-motivating statements (Miller & Rollnick 1991). These and other ways of responding are described in detail in Chapter 4.

A concept linked to importance is that of *wanting to change* or even *keenness* to change. The assessment question can be framed thus:

> *How do you feel **at the moment** about* [change]? *How much do you want to* [change]? *If 0 was 'not at all' and 10 was 'very much', what number would you give yourself?*

Scrutiny of these last two questions reveals that they approach the more general concept of readiness, or motivation to change. Patients respond well to questions about motivation. We have not suggested using this latter term in the assessment because, as noted above, some of our earlier work (see Rollnick et al 1997) led to theoretical confusion about the meaning of the term 'motivation'. Practitioners, however, can use whatever term they wish! In this particular assessment though, we are interested in penetrating the patients' feelings and views about the costs and benefits of change: its *personal value*, or whether it will, on balance, lead to an improvement in their lives, as distinct from the issue of their confidence to master the demands of this change.

Assess confidence

In keeping with the meaning of the term self-efficacy, we are interested here not in a general sense of confidence or self-esteem, but in confidence about mastering the various situations in which behavior change will be challenged. The most direct question we have found is:

*If you decided **right now** to* [change] *how confident do you feel about succeeding with this? If 0 was 'not confident' and 10 was 'very confident', what number would you give yourself?*

What to talk about next: importance or confidence?

The outcome of this assessment is sometimes clear. The patient has little concern about one dimension and the obvious difficulty lies with the other one. It is then a matter of deciding what strategy will help this person to either explore importance or build confidence. A menu of options within each dimension is provided in the next chapter.

Sometimes it is not clear, or both dimensions appear salient. Here one enters a labyrinth comprising the world of *Can I, should I, will I, won't I?*, often not merely connected to behavior change, but tied up with other personal matters:

I'd like to lose weight, but eating gives me such comfort. There's sometimes a hollow feeling in my stomach, when I get anxious or cross, the stress just gets too much. Then after eating so much I feel disgusted with myself. It will be really difficult to stop this.

Habits can be complex, and hard to change. Under circumstances like the above, practitioners clearly need to lower their sights if the contact time is brief. Being too ambitious is probably the biggest mistake to make, often taking the form of premature action talk, like *Why don't we try to take things one step at a time, and start with* .... Resistance is a likely outcome. One possibility is that the discussion returns to agenda setting, and moves onto another issue. If behavior change is to be talked about, a period of uncertainty is likely to prevail in which the practitioner should ultimately use the patient as the guide for deciding whether to focus on importance or confidence.

We suggest the following guidelines for deciding whether to focus on importance or on confidence. Practitioners should bear in mind, however, that there is no blueprint for decision making, only aids for what is often an intuitive judgment.

- If the importance level is depressed, focus on this if at all possible.
- Focus on the lower number, importance or confidence, particularly if there is a large discrepancy between them.
- If they are roughly equal, then start with importance.
- If they are both very low, then lower your sights. Were you wise to focus on behavior change in the first place? Consider the possibility that some other issue might be more relevant. Share this observation with the patient. Try to reach some agreement about exactly how the patient is feeling. Within each of the sections on importance and confidence below, we suggest that one option is to do little more beyond this assessment.

Is confidence easier to talk about than importance?

Many practitioners assume that confidence building is easier to talk about, perhaps because this is congruent with a culture of action-oriented professional practice in healthcare settings. This can even take the form of viewing motivational problems as confined to the issue of importance, as if confidence building is somehow free of these difficulties (see Chapter 2, p. 23). This can lead one into a trap: the former is viewed as complex, while the latter is viewed as a more simple practical matter of helping with strategies for improving confidence. Now, when talking about confidence building, one can get down to the real business of behavior change, apparently free of the delicate dance around the forces of resistance and motivation. Armed with this kind of understanding, a descent into advice-giving is usually just around the corner, and the response of the patient to suggestions about trying this or that action plan is predictable: *Yes, but I've tried that, and it doesn't work because ....* Motivational problems can arise when talking about either dimension, for example, *I could if I wanted to, but ...!* (importance issue), or *I want to but ...* (a confidence issue). There is no reason to believe that one is essentially simpler to talk about than the other. Ambivalence about change can surely arise because of concerns about either or both?

STRATEGY 2: ASSESS READINESS TO CHANGE

There can be situations where it is useful to assess readiness, either instead of or in addition to importance and confidence. It can be a useful platform for taking the discussion a step further. We tend to view this more global dimension as something to be aware of on an ongoing basis throughout the consultation, not necessarily something to be assessed. It often provides an explanation for resistance, if you overestimate the patient's general readiness to change (see Chapter 5).

Stage-based or continuum?

If you do want to assess readiness, should you do this using the notion of stages or that of a continuum? In the world of theory and psychometric assessment, this matter is still the subject of debate (see Sutton 1996, Budd and Rollnick 1996, Davidson 1998). It is not clear which approach is more useful to practitioners. We have heard good arguments either way. A stage-based assessment appears to be clear and simple for both practitioner and patient. For practitioners new to this construct, the notion of stages can be very useful. As Prochaska and DiClemente have repeatedly pointed out, many behavior change efforts have been restricted to an action-oriented approach when most patients are not at this stage in the first place (see DiClemente & Prochaska 1998). Use of stage designations can be good for highlighting this kind of problem.

How one responds to a stage-based assessment is crucial. We do not suggest that practitioners think of a patient's identified stage of change as being linked with a specific intervention, for the reasons described above (p. 60). Our starting point with a stage-based assessment would be to ask a patient why he or she is in one stage and not another. This would open up the conversation for the patient to describe whatever basis there is to his or her motivation to change. We suspect that the conversation will inevitably turn to importance or confidence. One can also use a stage-based assessment, particularly if it is in the form of a questionnaire, as a strategy for feeding back to the patient your understanding of how other people feel about change, using the principles for information exchange described in Chapter 5, and derived from the work of Miller and colleagues on the drinker's check-up (Miller et al 1988, Miller & Sovereign 1989). Thus, the expressed stage is used as the platform for letting the patient interpret the personal meaning of his or her views in relation to others.

On the other hand, we all know that people jump in and out of stages. In fact, although not wishing to stray too far into the realms of the philosophy of mind, it has occurred to us many times in consultations that patients have different 'voices' in their minds at any one time, representing different stages. This is particularly true for people designated as contemplators. A mood of concern and optimism about change can swing to one of defensiveness and defiance in a matter of seconds. Practitioners, for their part, can become part of this conflict. Speak to them in one way, for example in a slightly coercive manner, and a resisting precontemplator's voice will emerge. Speak to them in another way, and a more optimistic voice can emerge. Thus, the apparent stage of change 'in' the patient is the product of the relationship with the practitioner. This added complexity can render a stage-based assessment, particularly if viewed as a fixed, almost trait-like quality, oversimplified. It is for this reason that we find a continuum-based approach to assessment and strategy selection more fluid and easier to fit into a conversation.

Formal versus informal assessment

This assessment, like that of importance and confidence, can be done informally or explicitly. In the latter approach outlined below, we introduce a Readiness Rule, which we have found useful in clinical practice. Of course, there is nothing to stop a practitioner developing a similar practical tool divided into different stages or, indeed, built around the concepts of importance and confidence. Practitioners, like patients, have their preferences, and care should be taken not to view any piece of technology as comprising standard practice for all encounters.

In summary, people vary in their readiness to change their behavior: if you jump ahead of a patient, for example by giving advice when he or she is not ready to change, resistance will be the outcome, and your time will have been wasted. Your goal is to understand patients' degrees of readiness to change, and to help them move forward towards decision making, if they see this as worthwhile. Remember, that readiness to change fluctuates between and within consultations.

How not to do it

Any of these strategies will ensure that you are wrong about most patients, most of the time:

- Assume that the patient is or should be ready to change, and proceed accordingly. Give advice.
- Use an oversimplified and dichotomous model of behavior change, i.e. patients are either motivated to change, or not. Respond accordingly, and you will find that most are apparently not ready to change. There is not much you can do about that until the patient in question is really ready to change.
- Assume that the patient will or should do anything you say because you are the expert.
- Assume that all patients are 'intractable' pleasure seekers who have no interest at all in looking after their health.

Towards good practice

Be specific

Readiness to do what? Usually, but not always, one is talking about a specific behavior. It is useful to be clear about this, and if you are not sure, check this with the patient. For example, taking the case of eating, there is a difference between each of the following: readiness to talk about it, to change diet in general, to lose weight, to keep weight steady, to eat less fatty foods, to eat more fruit and vegetables, and so on. Each of these could be a useful topic for discussion (see Chapter 8, p. 189).

Assess readiness

Three assessment methods are noted below, using open questions, a numerical scaling method, and the *readiness rule*. The last of these is described in some detail, although it is important to note that these guidelines apply equally well to the two other methods of assessment. The assessment of readiness is a process, not an event, involving conversation and reflection.

The easiest method to use is to ask simple *open questions*, and then follow the patient's response carefully. For example:

How do you really feel about ——? How ready to change are you?

People differ quite a lot in how ready they are to change their ——. What about you?

Some people don't want to talk about drinking at all, others are unsure, and some don't mind at all. How do you feel about this?

One can also use a *numerical scaling* method, for example:

If 0 was 'not ready' and 10 was 'ready', what score would you give yourself?

Here one can follow the response with the kind of questions outlined in detail in Chapter 4, where a similar method is described for responding to the assessment of importance and confidence, for example:

You gave yourself a score of x. Why are you at x and not [a lower number]?

You gave yourself a score of x. What would have to happen for you to move up to [a higher number]?

A third method is to use something like the readiness rule (Fig. 3.4).

1. Introduce the assessment (the ruler or a line on a piece of paper). For example: *How ready to change [behavior] are you. Where are you on this ruler? Are you here [pointing to right-hand end], ready to change, are you more towards the middle, or the left-hand side?*
2. Elicit the patient's judgment. If this is hampered by lack of information, ask the patient if he or she would like more information. Remember that this task might generate quite a lot of discussion. Do not rush this process, as it is crucial to decision making.

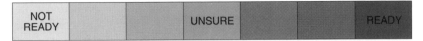

Figure 3.4   A readiness rule. Adapted from Stott et al 1995 Family Practice Vol 12 No 4 pp 413–416 Fig 2, Oxford University Press, with permission of the publisher.

Consider the next step

In general, if the patient appears unready, your only viable strategy might be to turn to information exchange. If there is some readiness to at least consider change, try to work out whether you need to assess importance or motivation. If this is obvious, then an appropriate strategy within either of these domains should be useful.

Watch the patient

Readiness to change fluctuates, particularly in the right-hand half of the continuum. Monitor this throughout the consultation. When people describe themselves as being on the right-hand end of the continuum, do not push them into decision making. Remember that the consultation does not have to end with them having gone through the gate saying something like, 'Yes, I'll definitely do something about it'. Even a decision to think about it can be a useful conclusion.

READINESS, IMPORTANCE AND CONFIDENCE

If you were to assess all three dimensions, which kind of patterns are likely to emerge? Another related question, and perhaps a more useful one, is to ask, at different degrees of readiness, what are the patterns which emerge on the other two dimensions? Researchers have looked at this second question, although this has taken the form of cross-sectional 'snapshots' of people's expectations at different stages, rather than prospective studies of how they change as they shift forward through the stages. It does appear that the shift from early stages of readiness to later ones is associated with clear shifts in the perceived importance of change, i.e. as one might expect, change is perceived as more important as one becomes increasingly ready (Rollnick et al 1996). There is apparently also a crossover effect in which the pros of change eventually outweigh the cons as people move through stages (Prochaska 1994). Confidence issues appear to become more salient in later stages, although the evidence for this thus far is incomplete (Davidson 1998, Rollnick 1998).

From a clinical vantage point, these observations are important. If someone's readiness is low, the chances are that it is importance which is the key issue. In the later stages of change, the person might be concerned about either importance or confidence. Indeed, one might even encounter a potentially bewildering overlap between importance and confidence in these later stages. It is in the melting pot of the contemplation stage, or to the right of the midway point on a readiness to change continuum, that the questions *Why should I?* and *How should I do it?* often collide.

Agenda setting and assessment of importance and confidence

Nurse: *Hello Mrs Brown. How are you?* (Checks immediate problems and concerns).

Mrs Brown: *I'm fine apart from being tired. The youngest boy's got a bit of a cough and I'm having to get up a couple of times a night so I'm not getting enough sleep just now.*

Nurse: *Do you want the doctor to see him?*

Mrs Brown: *No. Thanks, he's got cough medicine and I think he'll be OK in a day or two, but I'll bring him in at the end of the week if he doesn't improve.*

Nurse: *Yes, do, if you're at all concerned. So this appointment was to talk about your weight, wasn't it?* (Raises the issue)

Mrs Brown: *Yes. You wanted me to lose some weight and I've been trying to slim on and off for years.*

Nurse: *So you've tried dieting?*

Mrs Brown: *Yes, every diet you can name!*

Nurse: *We could either look again at diets, or look at how you could burn up more of the food you eat by being more active, or we could look at both.* (Invites patient to set agenda)

Mrs Brown: *I think I probably know more about calories and diets than the doctor does! But I've never really made any effort to do any exercise when I'm dieting. I might think about that.* (Patient sets agenda)

Nurse: *How do you feel about becoming more active? Is it something you want to do? How important is it to you right now?* (Informal assessment of importance)

Mrs Brown: *Well, when I was a girl I used to love sports – I was in the school hockey team and was never out of the swimming pool. Since the kids,*

I've let myself go a bit. I would like to feel fitter as well as losing some weight. I know I'd feel better about myself. I'd love to take the boys swimming now they're getting older too. (Patient gives information about her physical activity history and about how important it is to her to change)

Nurse: *So it's quite important to you?*

Mrs Brown: *Very, now I come to think about it, but I've no idea whether it's realistic. Swimming would be the place to start but I don't know how I'd find the time and I'm not sure I'd have the nerve to be seen in a swimming costume – the size I am now!*

Nurse: *So you want to do it but you don't feel all that confident about it? If you decided right now to start swimming regularly, how confident do you feel about succeeding? If 0 stands for 'not confident' and 10 stands for 'very confident', what number would you give yourself?* (Formal assessment of confidence)

Mrs Brown: *Less than 5 at the moment. Partly because of the time and partly because I'd feel self-conscious. Perhaps if there was a time in the middle of the day when the kids are at school and nursery and the pool is nice and quiet …? I don't know really.*

The nurse has structured the consultation clearly, but Mrs Brown has had space to express her own interests and concerns. Having clarified that it is important to her to lose weight, and to make physical activity a key behavior change towards this goal, it is obvious that confidence building should be the focus. Note that if you count the words in this dialog, the nurse says less than Mrs Brown. The nurse mainly asks questions and clarifies points. Mrs Brown is talking herself towards an action plan, so far without needing any advice.

REFERENCES

Budd R J, Rollnick S 1996 The structure of the readiness to change questionnaire: a test of Prochaska and DiClemente's transtheoretical model. British Journal of Health Psychology 1:365–376

Butler C C, Rollnick S, Cohen D, Russell I, Bachmann M, Stott N (in press) Motivational consulting versus brief advice for smokers in general practice: a randomised trial. British Journal of General Practice

Davidson R The transtheoretical model: a critical overview. 1998 In: Miller R W, Heather N (eds) Treating addictive behaviors, 2nd edn. Plenum, New York

de Shazer S, Berg I, Lipchick E, Nunnally E, Molnar A, Gingerich W, Weiner-Davies M 1986 Brief therapy: a focused solution development. Family Process 25:207–222

DiClemente C C, Prochaska J 1998 Toward a comprehensive, transtheoretical model of change: stages of change and addictive behaviors. In: Miller W R, Heather N (eds) Treating addictive behaviors, 2nd edn. Plenum, New York

Miller W R, Rollnick S 1991 Motivational interviewing: preparing people to change addictive behavior. Guilford Press, New York

Miller W R, Sovereign R 1989 The check-up: a model for early intervention in addictive behaviors. In Loberg T, Miller W R, Nathan P E, Marlatt G A (eds) Addictive behaviors: prevention and early intervention. Swets & Zeitlinger, Amsterdam

Miller W, Sovereign G, Krege B 1988 Motivational interviewing with problem drinkers: II. The drinker's check-up as a preventative intervention. Behavioural Psychotherapy 16:251–268

Powell T J, Enright S J 1990 Anxiety and stress management. Routledge, London

Prochaska J O 1994 Strong and weak principles for progressing from precontemplation to action on the basis of twelve problem behaviours. Health Psychology 13:47–51

Rollnick S 1998 Readiness, importance and confidence: critical conditions of change in treatment. In: Miller W R, Heather N (eds) Treating addictive behavior, 2nd edn. Plenum, New York

Rollnick S, Mason P 1992 Negotiating behavior change: a selection of strategies. Unpublished manual

Rollnick S, Morgan M, Heather N 1996 The development of a scale to measure outcome expectations of reduced consumption among excessive drinkers. Addictive Behaviours 21:377–387

Rollnick S, Butler C C, Stott N 1997 Helping smokers make decisions: the enhancement of brief intervention for general medical practice. Patient Education and Counseling 31:191–203

Stott N C H, Pill R M 1990 Advise yes, dictate no. Patients' views on health promotion in the consultation. Family Practice 7:125–131

Stott N C H, Rollnick S, Rees M, Pill R 1995 Innovation in clinical method: diabetes care and negotiating skills. Family Practice 12:413–418

Stott N C H, Rees M, Rollnick S, Pill R, Hackett P 1996 Professional responses to innovation in clinical method: diabetes care and negotiation skills. Patient Education and Counseling 29:67–73

Sutton S 1996 Can 'stages of change' provide guidance in the treatment of addictions? A critical examination of Prochaska and DiClemente's model. In: Edwards G, Dare C (eds) Psychotherapy, psychological treatments and the addictions. Cambridge University Press, Cambridge

4

Explore importance and build confidence

Maybe I will quit one day, maybe I won't. Giving up is not really a problem. I've done it before without any problem whatsoever. I enjoy smoking and it doesn't seem to be doing me any harm. I know I shouldn't

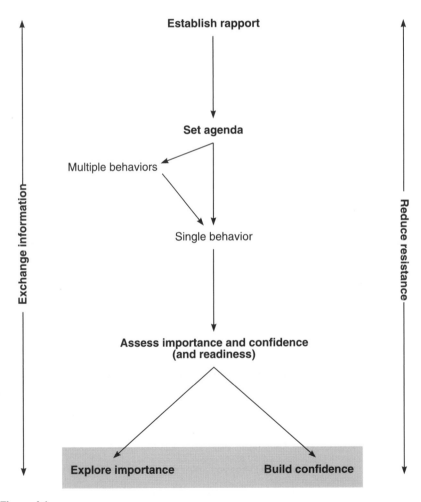

Figure 4.1

smoke in front of the children, especially little Anna with her bad chest. I don't suppose it sets a very good example. Still, my granny smoked 80 a day for 60 years and got run over by a bus while she was running across the road at the age of 85! I just enjoy smoking and it doesn't worry me.

Some patients attach a low importance to behavior change.

It's no good me trying to stop smoking. I know what you're saying is right. I ought to and I've tried lots of times but I've got no willpower. I last a couple of weeks and I'm back where I started.

I really can't see myself being able to remember to take this inhaler three times a day. It's easy to remember when my chest is bad. But when I feel better I just forget completely although I know it's important to prevent my asthma attacks. I'm just not organized enough to do it.

Sometimes people have so little confidence it doesn't seem worth them even trying (See Figure 4.1).

Box 4.1 Useful Questions

Explore importance

- *What would have to happen for it to become much more important for you to change?*
- *What would have to happen before you seriously considered changing?*
- *Why have you given yourself such a high score on importance?*
- *What would need to happen for your importance score to move up from x to y?*
- *What stops you moving up from x to y?*
- *What are the good things about ... [current behavior]. What are some of the less good things about ... [current behavior]? (Alternative: Things you like and dislike...)*
- *What concerns do you have about ... [current behavior]?*
- *If you were to change, what would it be like?*
- *Where does this leave you now? (when you want to ask about change in a neutral way)*

Build confidence

- *What would make you more confident about making these changes?*
- *Why have you given yourself such a high score on confidence?*
- *How could you move up higher, so that your score goes from x to y?*
- *How can I help you succeed?*
- *Is there anything you found helpful in any previous attempts to change?*
- *What have you learned from the way things went wrong last time you tried?*
- *If you were to decide to change what might your options be? Are there any ways you know about that have worked for other people?*
- *What are some of the practical things you would need to do to achieve this goal? Do any of them sound achievable?*
- *Is there anything you can think of that would help you feel more confident?*

Having assessed the importance of change for a patient and his or her confidence to put plans to change into action (see Chapter 3), you reach a critical junction. You need to decide where to go next, and which of these two dimensions to focus on. This chapter summarizes a selection of strategies for working within either dimension.

TWO MENUS OF STRATEGIES

For each of these topics, importance and confidence, we have constructed a menu of strategies. These are listed on pages 77 and 96. Which ones to use depends very much on the circumstances, your aspirations and the needs of the patient.

The delicate dance

In moving both within and between these dimensions, the practitioner will require all the skill and deftness of a dancer leading a partner through a sequence of movements, simultaneously leading and being led, keenly alert to subtle threats to the synchrony of the partnership. Resistance from the partner is not met by force, but by transforming the movement in a constructive direction, if at all possible. No amount of dedicated adherence to the strategies described below will be effective if this state of mind is absent. The strategies are merely aids to avoiding collision, like the steps one learns in a dancing class.

A certain degree of relaxation is required to maintain this spirit in the consultation. As we have noted earlier in this book, we have found it useful to develop a *committed* but *curious* state of mind when talking about behavior change. There is no sense in which you can be expected to have all the answers. Indeed, you must believe that these lie mostly within the patient.

OVERLAPPING OF IMPORTANCE AND CONFIDENCE

The possibility of importance and confidence issues being interconnected was discussed briefly in the last chapter. In earlier stages of readiness there is often a clear distinction between them: importance is usually low, and is probably the dimension on which you need to focus. In later stages of readiness, however, the perceived benefits and costs of change tend to hinge upon confidence issues. For example, many overweight patients have no doubt about the value of change, but because they have low levels of confidence, the perceived value of change is depressed accordingly. One of the obstacles they anticipate which devalues change is an inability to control their eating in different situations.

Thus when working with strategies applicable to fairly high levels of importance, the distinction between importance and confidence can become blurred, not with every patient, but certainly with some of them. Use of strategies like *exploring concerns* or *a hypothetical look over the fence* can thus involve discussion of confidence issues as well. Learning to move between these two dimensions in the melting pot of later stages of readiness is certainly a challenge. If you get confused, ask the patient, since your task is not to solve problems, but to encourage patients to do this themselves.

TASK: EXPLORE IMPORTANCE
The strategies

Some of the strategies for working on importance are best used at fairly high levels of this dimension (i.e. with scores above 5/10 on the formal assessment). This applies particularly to *exploring concerns*; for example, if a patient does not see change as particularly important, and you use a strategy like exploring concerns, you could be in trouble! The patient will say, 'What concerns?'. The same logic applies to the last strategy on the list below. Others are safer or more widely applicable at all levels of importance, for example, *scaling questions* and *examining pros and cons*. The strategies below are thus presented in ascending order of suitability to patients, from lower to higher levels of perceived importance.

Your use of words to describe different degrees of concern about a behavior can be critical. If a patient says, *My drinking is sometimes a problem*, and you use the word *alcoholic* you could be in trouble. If you give people a chance to talk, they will use a variety of words about change. You should watch out for these and match them as far as possible. Many of the strategies below start with a leading question which implies knowledge of how concerned the patient is about a behavior. Sometimes, however, one does not get a lead from the patient, and one has to take a deep breath and see what happens.

We have noticed that, if one imagines a continuum of importance, from 0 to 10, different words are suitable at different points along this continuum. The words *What is it you don't like about ...?* is the safest bet, applicable for most people, as long as the level of reported importance is not zero. In ascending order, the following terms are appropriate as the level of importance gets higher: *dislikes* or *less good things* (2–3/10 or above), *concerns* (6/10 or above), *difficulty* or *problem* (7–8/10 or above). If you use one of the latter terms with low levels of importance, the damaged rapport will be your responsibility to repair!

A menu of strategies

Five strategies are described in this section, all of them options for exploring importance:

1. Do little more
2. Scaling questions
3. Examine the pros and cons
4. Explore concerns about the behavior
5. A hypothetical look over the fence.

The range of strategies for exploring importance is best viewed as a menu from which you select one to suit your needs. Indeed, we suggest that if you have time for development work, you adapt these and construct new ones more appropriate to your client group.

Care should be taken not to view these strategies as techniques applied *to* or *on* patients. If this happens it is an indication of detachment which we presume will damage rapport. The strategies are simply ways of structuring a purposeful conversation. Their specificity should also not be misunderstood: this is intended as a guide, as a concrete reference point which we know is likely to minimize resistance. As noted from the outset, creative adaptation, not slavish adoption, should be the goal.

STRATEGY 1: DO LITTLE MORE

If a patient's level of perceived importance is markedly low, particularly if accompanied by a low level of confidence, it might be advisable to close discussion of behavior change and either turn to a more important issue or end the consultation. How this is done is important. You could leave the patient feeling downhearted or even reluctant to come back and see you. Consider saying something like:

> *Perhaps now is not the right time to talk about this? How do you feel?*

> *You say you are unsure about what to do. I do not want to push you into a decision, it's really up to you. I suggest that you take your time to think about it. I have met other people who have felt just like you do. Some, for good reasons of their own, decide not to do anything for the time being. Others do the opposite, and make the change. You will be the best judge of when is the right time to consider change. Is there some other issue that feels more important to you?*

Whatever you do, acknowledge the uncertainty, do not just leave the patient hanging in the air. If you are not sure what to do, ask the patient. For example, he or she might want to talk about it again on another occasion.

Many practitioners, faced with this situation are tempted to take a deep breath and simply provide *information*, seeing it as their professional responsibility to at least inform the patient of existing or potential risks. If this does not damage rapport, the approach seems understandable and justified.

STRATEGY 2: SCALING QUESTIONS

This involves using a set of questions designed to understand and encourage the patient to explore the whole question of the personal value or importance of change in more detail. It is based on the numerical assessment described in Chapter 3 (see de Shazer et al 1986), although it can also be adapted in non-numerical form. Typically, having elicited a numerical judgment of importance, the set of simple questions noted below can open up a very productive discussion in which the patient is doing most of the talking and is thinking hard about change (see Rollnick et al 1997).

How not to do it

Having obtained a numerical judgment of perceived importance, change the subject, or push the person too hard in an unrealistic way. Show no curiosity, only purposefulness.

> *So you would give this topic 5/10 for importance. Fine. Now, how would you actually go about giving up smoking? We've had a lot of success lately with nicotine patches.*

Towards good practice

You have already conducted an assessment of how important it is to the patient to change and you have in mind a given level, ideally a number (see Chapter 3, p. 63), although this is not essential.

- Ensure that the pace of the discussion is slowed down, and develop a genuine curiosity to know how this person really feels. You should *listen* to the answers to your questions, using techniques like reflection and other simple open questions to help patients express themselves as fully as possible. Your attention should not be on your own thought processes (e.g. *What should I ask next?*), but as much as possible on the meaning of what the person is saying. Trust the process and the patient.
- Watch carefully for resistance, because this is a signal that you are going too far.
- Ask either or both of the following questions, and then follow them on with other open questions or reflective listening statements.

1. 'Why so high?'

This kind of question should not be asked if the patient's rating of perceived importance is too low, i.e. around 1–2/10, for obvious reasons!

Ask why he or she had scored a given number and not a lower number.

You said that it was fairly important to you personally to change
[behavior]. Why have you scored 6 and not 1?

The answers amount to positive reasons for change, or in the jargon of
motivational interviewing, a series of *self-motivational statements* (see Miller
1983, Miller & Rollnick 1991). For example:

I am at 6 and not 1 because I cannot go on like this forever. An obvious
response is simply to ask *Why?*

Your task is now to elicit the range of reasons why the person wants to
change. The pace should be slow, and simple open questions can be very
useful here. If the answers are obvious, then elicit them and move on. If
more complex, then take your time trying to understand all the ramifications.

2. 'How can you go higher?'

A second kind of question moves in the opposite direction, up the scale
from the number given by the person. For example: *You gave yourself a score*
of 6. So it's fairly important for you to change [behavior]. *What would have to*
happen for your score to move up from 6 to 9? or: *How could you move up from 6*
to 8 or even 9? or: *What stops you moving up from 6 or 7?* Note that one can ask
about either *your score* or just *you*. The second method often feels like the
better one.

An illustration

Here is an example of dialog which illustrates that the key challenge for the
practitioner is to carefully follow the patient's response, with further questions and reflective listening statements. In this example the practitioner
starts with the first kind of question described above (*Why so high?*), and
then simply follows the responses of the patient. It was not necessary to
move on to using the second kind of question (*How can you go higher?*). The
conversation flowed quite naturally into that territory, i.e. what would
make the person more motivated. Note how the use of a new strategy
involves being quite directive to begin with.

Practitioner: [A few minutes into the consultation. Decides that the
patient will respond to a quick assessment of importance and
confidence] *How do you really feel about taking more exercise? If 0 was*
'not important to you at the moment', and 10 was 'very important', what
number would you give yourself?

Patient: [a short silence] *About 6.*

Practitioner: *And if you did decide now to take more exercise, how confident are you that you would succeed? If 0 was 'not confident' and 10 was 'very confident', what number would you give yourself?*

Patient: *About 8.*

Practitioner: *So if you decided to do it, you feel fairly confident, but you are not sure how important it is for you right now.*

Patient: *Well yes, that's about right.*

Practitioner: *You said it was fairly important for you, a score of about 6. Why did you give yourself 6, and not 1?*

Patient: [initial silence] *I am at 6 and not 1 because the last time I got into my old swimming routine, it was great – but such hard work. Now that I have had a heart attack I guess I should go back to it.*

Practitioner: *It will be good for you.*

Patient: *Well that's what you people always say!*

Practitioner: *But you're not so sure.*

Patient: *No. How do you know my heart won't take too much strain?*

Practitioner: *You're worried that swimming will damage your heart.*

Patient: *Not worried, terrified.*

Practitioner: *How exactly do you see this happening?*

Patient: *Well, I feel so sick right now, like my life hangs on a thread. I feel scared walking to the toilet sometimes.*

Practitioner: *You just don't know what's going to happen.*

Patient: *Yes, that's right.*

Practitioner: [Decides to use information exchange. Becomes more directive.] *Have you ever had a good talk about what happens in the heart after a heart attack?*

Patient: *Yes, sort of, but I don't understand…*

In this example, the consultation did not linger for too long in the response to the first kind of scaling question, *Why did you score 6 and not 1?* No other reasons for scoring 6 were elicited, for example, by asking something like, *What else makes you score 6 and not 1?* The patient's feelings about this seemed obvious. Sometimes the perceived benefits and costs are less clear; this is often the case with talk about drinking, when it can be worthwhile to linger longer at this task.

Note also that the practitioner could have returned to the structure provided by the scaling question on a number of occasions, e.g. *So your fear of damaging your heart is stopping you taking more exercise. Were it not for this, what score would you give yourself for wanting to get more exercise?* In this example, however, the scaling method was used as a springboard, not as a scaffold for the entire conversation. In other situations it can be very useful to go back to the scale and the numbers.

You might wonder about the outcome of this kind of discussion. Where should it lead? It is unwise to generalize about this, because it depends on the unique needs of the individual. The point is that simply talking about the importance dimension can help to clarify things. It might or it might not lead to firm talk about change. It is best to follow the patient. If the discussion ends without action talk, simply summarize what has been said, offer whatever future support you can, and leave it at that. The aim of the consultation is not to get agreement or a decision to change. Exploring importance is just that – exploration.

STRATEGY 3: EXAMINE THE PROS AND CONS

Unlike the strategy just described, use of this one does not have to be based on an explicit assessment of perceived importance. It is sometimes completely obvious that the importance of behavior change is an issue, and the only challenge is to decide what strategy to use. If it is preceded by an assessment, this strategy is ideal when the score is around 5/10 on the scale. At 1/10 the patient might not perceive any costs associated with the behavior at all.

Ambivalence about the value of change

One aspect of the ambivalence conflict (see Miller & Rollnick 1991) focuses on the costs and benefits of both staying the same and change. A conflict like that described in Table 4.1 might arise. Whichever way the person turns, there are costs and benefits associated with each option, change or no change. This has been termed a double approach–avoidance conflict.

The different ways in which people experience this kind of conflict are not understood well enough. Certainly the experience embraces both psychological and social dimensions. In the addictions field, it has been well documented by Orford (1985). From excessive drinking, through gambling, to forms of sexual promiscuity, the intense battle between episodes of indulgence and restraint can render a person confused, elated, guilty, depressed, optimistic, and often enmeshed in conflict with others. It is therefore not surprising that alternatives to direct persuasion like motiva-

Table 4.1 Ambivalence

Someone facing the apparent need to change their diet might feel thus:

No change	Change
Costs	**Costs**
Feel ugly and unattractive	Will have to think about what to eat all the time
Difficult to buy nice clothes	Will have to give up my favorite junk foods
Greater risk of heart disease and diabetes	Healthy food is often expensive
Can't run around easily with the children	
Benefits	**Benefits**
Don't have to think about what to eat, can eat with the family	Feel good about achieving it
Can eat the food I really like	May feel fitter and be healthier
	If I lose weight I will feel more attractive and confident and be able to buy nice clothes
	Will be able to be more active

tional interviewing were first developed in the addictions field (see Miller 1983). The potential for conflict with a counselor is great. Within a few minutes a patient's mood can swing from defiance to remorse, from agreement about a problem to apparent denial of one.

Dimensions of the dilemma

The example cited above does not necessarily describe someone in the throes of a severe addictive problem, or what Orford (1985) called an *excessive appetite*. It could be a much more common dilemma. Mood swings might not be so severe and there is no reason to believe that overweight or even obese people walk around in a state of severe conflict. We simply do not know enough about how people facing behavior change feel. Clinical experience tells us that, among the people seen in healthcare settings where behavior change is discussed, the nature and extent of the conflict vary considerably. This variation occurs on a number of dimensions.

One of the most striking variations is in the *breadth* of the conflict. Some people truly are faced with the kind of multifaceted conflict described in Table 4.1. Others appear to be very uncertain about change not because they are in conflict about the status quo, but because one major issue or perceived cost of change predominates over all else. An example would be a back pain sufferer who would very much like to become more active, but who feels reluctant to do some simple exercises because of a fear of causing further damage.

There is also variation in people's *awareness* of the conflict, and whether they have spoken about it before. Smokers, it seems, are usually aware of the competing costs and benefits, excessive drinkers generally less so. Some patients have never spoken about their feelings and views before, and leave one feeling privileged to be hearing an account for the first time. Yet we all know patients for whom this is all familiar territory, almost to the point where they are ready and waiting for the practitioner to open up this little black box. They know the contents, and they are ready with the answers that allow them to avoid consideration of change at this point in their lives.

An interesting dimension is the degree of *emotional intensity* involved. This varies across individuals and behaviors. Generalization would be unwise, as would a conclusion about whether it is better to encourage patients to explore these issues on an emotional or a cognitive level. Sometimes the emotional expression of ambivalence can feel confusing for patients, and it is the articulation on a more cognitive level which seems clearer, more conscious and more helpful. The opposite can also be true. It is probably best to let the patient be one's guide here, paying careful attention to resistance at all times. We have also found that as the patient makes a decision to change and ambivalence is resolved (at least temporarily), this is often accompanied by an emotional reaction. The person sighs deeply or even becomes upset. This can be most constructive, although the patient will obviously need commitment from the practitioner to look after him or her in an appropriate way.

Finally, there is often a distinction between short and long-term consequences, with the former having a more powerful effect on decision making than the latter.

In summary then, this aspect of ambivalence is not like an accountant's balance sheet, rigid and rational, consistent in structure. It is an individual conflict about the *personal* value of change, often riddled with unique perceptions and contradictions. As such, there are few grounds for dogmatism and generalization about its content.

How not to do it

Argue strongly for change by either: (1) telling the patient about the costs of continuing with current behavior; or (2) telling the patient about the advantages of change. Use of either of these strategies will almost certainly ensure that the patient will present the opposing argument. Motivation not to change will be reinforced, the patient will feel coerced, and you will probably feel frustrated. You will probably conclude that the patient is not motivated to change.

> Practitioner: *If you continue being so inactive your weight is going to keep going up and your risk of a heart attack is really quite high. I know you would feel much better in yourself if you did more and were fitter.*

> Patient: *But I'm far too busy to waste time going to gyms or running in circles round the park. One of my colleagues had a heart attack when he was out jogging last year and that put a lot of us off, I can tell you! I don't think exercise has anything to do with my weight anyway. We've always been big in my family.*

Table 4.2 Balance Sheet

No change	Change
Costs	**Costs**
Benefits	**Benefits**

Towards good practice

This strategy is best used in the consulting room. However, if time is short, you can ask the patient to do the work at home, using a blank copy of the balance sheet presented in Table 4.2.

Introduce the strategy: ask the patient

This strategy can take as little as 5–7 minutes to use. If you have more time, then use it, and let the patient explain things as fully as possible. The most important first step is to ask the patient whether he or she would like to examine the pros and cons. For example:

> *Would you like to spend a few minutes talking about your —— looking at what you like and don't like about it?*

or

> *Sometimes it can be helpful to examine the pros and cons of —— Would you like to spend a few minutes doing this, or would you prefer not to?*

Another approach is to present the balance sheet to the patient, for example:

> *Here is a drawing which might help us. You can see that, for all people who are unsure about change, there are **pros** and **cons** of staying the same [the present behavior], and then there's the other side, there are usually **pros** and **cons** of change as well. Have you ever thought about it like this? Would you like to spend a few minutes talking about it?*

Use of words is important here. The most common mistake is to use needlessly complicated words like 'costs' and 'benefits'. Even the use of 'advantages' and 'disadvantages' can be difficult for some patients; 'pros' and 'cons' are usually acceptable; we have used 'good things' and 'less good things' below. If possible, the use of 'like' and 'don't like' are ideal. Be careful also not to use words like 'problem' or 'concern' unless the patient has used them. They often imply a greater degree of concern than felt by the patient and can generate needless resistance, particularly with those who are less motivated to change.

One key decision is whether to focus on the pros and cons of continuing with the current behavior pattern, or pros and cons of changing. Note that the content of one side of the divide is often a mirror image of the other and that the distinction often breaks down in conversation with patients. Thus talk about cons of smoking (e.g. feeling unhealthy) will quite naturally evolve into talk about pros of change (feeling fitter). However, we suggest that you take the following rough guidelines into account. Start with the current behavior if:

- You don't know the patient very well.
- The patient seems unclear about the issues or has not had the chance to talk about them in a non-threatening environment.
- The patient is some distance from the preparation stage, i.e. is not actively thinking about change
- He or she feels ashamed about the behavior.

Examine the pros and cons

As noted above, there are two ways of examining the pros and cons, either to look at the *current behavior*, or *change*. The balance sheet visual aid is designed to help you and the patient work together. Beware, however: visual aids can get in the way of communicating with the patient. This depends on how you use them. We suspect that as practitioners become more skilled, so their need for visual aids diminishes.

The pros and cons of the current behavior Your role is to provide structure, listen carefully, and then summarize at the end. The patient's role is to explain to you how he or she really feels. Start with the positive, which will help with rapport building and place the behavior in a normal context. This can be a shock in some situations, particularly where the patient believes that the behavior is a problem. You can deal with this in a quite straightforward way, by explaining that there must be benefits from the activity or behavior, otherwise he or she would not be doing it. This is important for you to understand.

1 Ask a question like:
   What are the good things about [the behavior]?
   Elicit these, and summarize if necessary. Your role here is simply to
   understand. Try not to ask questions that do not have a direct bearing
   on this picture and its meaning. Simple open questions can be very
   useful, for example, *Why is this? In what way? How exactly does this affect*
   you?
2 Then ask a question like:
   What are the less good things about [the behavior]?
   Elicit these, one by one, taking as much time as possible; use simple
   open questions to understand exactly what the patient does not like
   about the behavior, for example, *What don't you like about——?* or *How*
   does this affect you?
3 Summarize both sides of the no change position, as succinctly as
   possible, with the same words as those used by the patient. This is a
   simple skill, but it does require practice. One needs to do at least
   two things at the same time: listen very carefully, and remember
   the exact key words used by the patient to describe the pros and
   cons.

The pros and cons of change This is useful if you think that the patient is
ready to look over the 'other side of the fence'.

1 Ask a question like
   What are the good things about change? Elicit these and summarize, if
   necessary.
2 Then ask a question like
   What are the less good things about change? Elicit these, slowly and
   carefully.
3 Summarize both sides of the change position, as succinctly as possible,
   using the patient's own terminology.

Reminders

- The goal of the consultation is not to have the patient say, *Yes, thanks, I*
  am going to change. It is to help the person to *think* about change. The
  matter does not have to be resolved in your consultation.
- Resistance can arise if you overestimate the personal value that a patient
  attaches to change.
- Patient resistance will be lowered if the practitioner's goal is simply to
  explore the importance of change, to elicit the key issues, not to provide
  them. The strategy is designed to help with this process.
- Remember that when a patient talks about the less good things or the
  things he or she does not like about a behavior, this is not equivalent to
  his or her concerns about it. *Concern* has a stronger emotional

connotation, which has been avoided in the strategy described above. If you ask someone who is not very ready to change about concerns, he or she might ask you, 'What concerns?' So too, for the same reason, be careful not to use the word 'problem' in this kind of discussion. However, most patients are able to express what they like or do not like about a behavior. Asking about concerns can be very useful, if the patient is more ready to change. This is the next strategy on the list.

STRATEGY 4: EXPLORE CONCERNS ABOUT THE BEHAVIOR

This strategy focuses solely upon the costs of the current behavior or situation. One can only use it, with its emphasis on the word 'concern', if the patient *appears* concerned. Misjudgment of this, i.e. overestimating the level of concern, will result in resistance. Otherwise it is ideal for helping the patient to take time to express exactly what the issues are. Its use will automatically generate self-motivating statements (Miller & Rollnick 1991). This strategy was developed in health promotion consultations with heavy drinkers, as a brief derivative of one of the main tasks of motivational interviewing (see Rollnick et al 1992). It focuses on the one side of the ambivalence diagram in Table 4.1, i.e. on concerns about the *current behavior*.

Of course, one could use this strategy to examine concerns about *change* as well.

How not to do it

Tell the patient what he or she ought to be concerned about and frighten him or her with horrible stories about what may happen if he or she does not change.

One in three smokers dies as a direct result of their smoking. Lung disease is a particularly horrible and frightening way to die. If I could take you now onto one of the surgical wards and introduce you to some of the lung cancer patients I guarantee you would take this more seriously.

Towards good practice

Ask about concerns

Two principles guide the use of this strategy: First, the patient, not the practitioner, expresses the concerns; and second, once the patient has reached the end, the practitioner asks some key questions about the possibility of change. **Your role** is to provide structure, listen carefully, and then summarize at the end. **The patient's role** is to explain to you how he or she really feels. To start off, either of the following two questions would be useful:

What concerns you the most about your [the behavior]?

or

What concerns do you have about [the behavior]?

Then simply follow the patient's description, attempting to understand exactly why he or she feels this way, under what circumstances, and so on. Take your time. Go through any other concerns he or she might have. Exchange information if appropriate, but try not to wander off task. Your role is to help the patient paint a picture of exactly why he or she is concerned. Then, summarize these concerns for the patient.

Ask about the next step

Ask the patient about the next step. Do this in a gentle and non-confrontational way, for example: *Where does this leave you now?* This kind of question is deliberately phrased in neutral terms. The patient can either move towards or away from a decision to change. A question which explicitly asks about change can be useful, but carries the risk of the patient feeling pushed too far.

Using a diary

Taking a realistic look at current behavior can increase motivation to change. Keeping a diary for a day or a week can be a useful way of understanding behavior and planning change. A patient who sees herself as a moderate drinker might be surprised by the number of glasses poured from the wine box, or the number of beer cans taken from the refrigerator. Similarly, someone who believes he is a healthy eater might underestimate the number of packets of crisps and other snacks eaten between meals. In summary, diary keeping clarifies when, how much, and in what context the behavior occurs.

It is less helpful to impose diaries upon patients: this should form part of a joint decision to examine the behavior in question. Care should be taken to establish a realistic time frame for keeping the diary which seems manageable to the patient.

Keeping a diary can serve other purposes, for example, in monitoring progress, once the patient has decided to change.

STRATEGY 5: A HYPOTHETICAL LOOK OVER THE FENCE

This is yet another way of examining the implications of behavior change. We have not developed it in any depth because its application seems mostly to be a simple repetition of one half of the pros and cons strategy described above, that which concerns *change*. It is highlighted here as a separate strategy mainly because of the way in which it is introduced to the patient, and because of the *hypothetical tone of the conversation as a whole*. It is best used at relatively high levels of perceived importance, i.e. at levels of the numerical equivalent of 7/10 or more, although this judgment is based on clinical speculation alone.

At the risk of stating the obvious, the higher the level of perceived importance, the more someone will be thinking about change, about what it might be like on the other side of the fence. However, even at these high levels, change can be difficult to talk about. We think this is because as the patient's overall readiness increases so he or she quite naturally has an almost simultaneous urge to back off. You ask about change, even in the form of an open-ended question like, 'How do you feel about change?' and they articulate the arguments against it. Sometimes this arises from a genuine desire to express concerns about change, which must be listened to, and certainly not argued against with a 'Yes, but …' response from the practitioner. At other times, however, one gets the feeling that this is merely a 'back-off' voice, repeating well-worn private arguments for staying the same. To gauge the difference between these two possible reasons for expressing concern about change can be very difficult.

It may be possible to lift both oneself and the patient out of this confusion by deliberately making the discussion hypothetical. This avoids the risk of a patient feeling threatened and using this 'back-off' voice. Both parties are taking a detached and curious look at what would happen. The patient is free to roam and speculate, without any pressure to make a decision in the consultation.

The opening sequence in the example below is one way of introducing this strategy. The exchange which follows highlights the tone of the discussion: this is explicitly curious and hypothetical throughout, and then ends with a reassurance that the conversation was not meant to push the patient towards change, only to encourage open discussion about it.

The overlap between importance and confidence issues is highlighted in the use of this strategy, particularly when it is used at fairly high levels of importance: what can tilt the balance in favor of change and make it feel more worthwhile is a clear vision of being able to achieve it. In this sense, *this strategy is suited to dealing with both importance and confidence issues*. It is placed here merely as a matter of convenience.

An example of a hypothetical look over the fence

Practitioner: *So you are not sure that it's a good idea to try to change your diet.*

Patient: *That's right.*

Practitioner: *Why don't we just imagine for a moment that you **did** make this change. How would you feel?*

Patient: *Not very excited* [laughs].

Practitioner: *You fear that you might get less enjoyment from food.*

Patient: *Exactly, yes, because I enjoy fried food.*

Practitioner: *You would have to deprive yourself.*

Patient: *Sometimes I would, yes, but would I have to stop fried foods altogether?*

Practitioner: *I'm not sure. I imagine that you might have quite a lot of freedom, to start slowly, to cut back a little, to find other foods that you like. You would have to decide what's best for you.*

Ethical reminder

It is when dealing with the importance dimension that you can often run into ethical difficulties. You might very much want the patient to change, and you unwittingly push him or her towards this. Perhaps even worse, you consciously use a subtle 'technique' for motivating change. To do this would be to violate the spirit of this kind of negotiation. Here are suggestions for protecting yourself and the patient:

- Be honest with the patient about what you are planning.
- Watch for resistance. If you are going further than the patient wants, he or she will resist.
- Understand the patient's point of view. Empathy is your protection. Let the patient be your guide.
- 'If in doubt, leave it out.' There might be very good reasons not to change.

A case example

Practitioner: *So, it's not very important to you, right now, to cut down your drinking? On a scale of 1–10 you said you would only give it a 4. You obviously enjoy a drink. Tell me some more about how it fits into a typical day for you.*

Patient: *Well, I only drink in the evenings. I've never been much of a lunchtime drinker. Most days I have a few beers in the club after work and then get a take-away on the way home. Often I'll have a whiskey as a nightcap while I watch some late night television.* (This is a very much shortened version of the Typical Day strategy described in Chapter 3.)

Practitioner: *So what is it you enjoy about a drink in the club after work?* (Elicits the pros of the current behavior)

Patient: *It helps me unwind and there's a regular crowd in there to have a laugh with. It passes the time too. Since I've been on my own I'm not so keen to go back to an empty house.*

Practitioner: *I can see that. And the nightcap?*

Patient: *That's partly habit and partly to make sure I sleep well.*

Practitioner: *I can see that there are lots of good things for you about drinking. Are there any not so good things?* (Elicits cons or self-motivating statements)

Patient: *Well, it takes up all my spare cash but as far as I'm concerned that doesn't matter as long as I'm enjoying myself.*

Practitioner: [senses a little resistance so backs off instead of asking directly about any other cons] *So, it helps you relax, pass the time and sleep well. You're not concerned that it takes up your spare cash because you enjoy it* (summarizes). *So why did you rate it as high as 4? Perhaps it's not even a 4 just now?* (Why so high?)

Patient: *Maybe not. Although a couple of the lads in the club have cut down lately on their doctor's advice. I'm fit as a fiddle but it did make me wonder whether I might be doing myself some damage without knowing it. I wouldn't want to make myself ill and I'd think twice if I thought I was.* (Unasked, gives a response to 'what would have to happen for you to seriously consider changing?') *How would I know if I was doing myself any harm? There isn't any way of knowing I suppose?*

Thus there is an opportunity to go on to exchange information, perhaps explore concerns about health related to the drinking and consider the pros of change.

TASK: BUILD CONFIDENCE

A patient was recently heard to say something which seemed like an echo of so many other consultations: *I need to lose weight. I understand why. I know what to do, and why I should do it. But tell me, why is it that I have so little moti-vation?* Some patients really want to change. It is important to them to do so. However, they feel pessimistic about the success of such a venture. The remainder of this chapter describes strategies for building confidence to succeed. These strategies provide a framework for something which is per-vasive in medical consultations and counseling sessions: helping people with practical solutions to their difficulties, building their confidence so that that they leave the discussion thinking, 'Yes, I can do that'. The fre-quency with which this activity occurs lies in sharp contrast to the absence of teachable strategies for improving its effectiveness (a similar situation to that other pervasive activity in consultations, information exchange; see Chapter 5). It could be argued that we do not need such strategies because we know how to do it: we give them good advice (see Chapter 2). One has only to observe oneself or other consultations to see how readily such talk can descend into an unconstructive dialog. It is a simple activity to concep-tualize, apparently, but difficult to succeed with. All too often, the patient says, 'Yes, but I've tried that and it doesn't work because...'

Self-efficacy: a useful concept

This concept can be misunderstood. It can appear like a piece of psycholog-ical jargon. However, once stripped down to essentials, it provides a useful bridge between the person and the social world in which he or she has to make changes to his or her behavior.

Self-efficacy refers to a person's confidence in his or her ability to make a specific change in behavior. This will vary across situations. For example, a smoker might feel very confident about resisting temptation to smoke at work, but less so when socializing with friends, and so on.

Self-efficacy is different from self-esteem, which is a more general sense of well-being that a person has about him- or herself and the life he or she leads. Bandura's (1977) social learning theory is based on the idea, well supported by a lot of research, that feelings of high self-efficacy are very important, and that it is in the world of doing, and watching others making changes, that people are successful; not just in the world of talking about doing, as occurs in the consulting room. This accords with clinical experi-ence: we know we are talking about most important matters with patients, i.e their confidence to make changes, yet we have to bear the frustration of being one step removed from the world in which the patient's ability is to be tested. We all know patients who say, *Yes, I know what I have to do, but I just can't succeed. I keep failing.* Bandura's work points to the importance not of some mysterious quality called willpower, but of levels of skill and ability, and actually working on changes in the real world.

For practitioners, the following practical guidelines can be derived from the work of Bandura and others (see, for example, Egan 1994):

- Self-efficacy is not an all-or-none quality. Since it varies across situations, one can provide encouragement and praise for those situations where it is high, and help the person look at different approaches for improving self-efficacy in situations where he or she feels less confident.
- Doing is the best way to enhance self-efficacy. Build as many bridges as you can between the consulting room and the patient's everyday life (e.g. bringing a partner to the next consultation, returning for brief meetings, keeping records).
- People need to have skills to succeed. Sometimes these lie dormant; sometimes they need to be built up. They are seldom either entirely present or totally absent.
- Feedback should be provided about deficiencies in performance, not deficiencies in the person (Egan 1994).
- People learn by modeling themselves on others, hence the value of talking about friends and patients who have succeeded, attending self-help groups, and so on.

The problem of low self-esteem

A more general feeling of low self-esteem and helplessness often underlies poor self-efficacy to make more specific changes. Furthermore, what manifests as a psychological 'problem' of low self-esteem often has strong social origins:

> *There's no chance of finding a job. So I can't move out of the damp flat. I haven't got the money to enjoy myself, and every time I try to change I fail. Now you say I must get my weight down.*

The strategies described below are not meant to be counseling strategies for dealing directly with low self-esteem and helplessness. Rather, they deal with more specific changes in self-efficacy about behavior change. Sometimes, however, you will find that *if* you can encourage someone to look at small changes, and if that person succeeds, these changes often have a bearing on gradually improving self-esteem. If not, simply acknowledging the way a person feels can start off a process of reversal of low self-esteem, particularly if you can offer further support.

Goals, strategies and targets

We use different terms to describe people's efforts to change behavior. Goals, strategies and targets are among the most widely used. Without wishing to become immersed in precise definitions, it can be useful to note the way in which the use of terms like these vary from the general to the specific. They can be likened to signposts on a journey. This might start with talk about a general *goal* or outcome being aimed at, which provides an answer to the question, *What change would you like to make?* Usually this refers to behavior change, although the goal of losing weight provides an interesting exception: losing weight is an outcome of behavior change rather than a behavior as such.

The journey often continues with talk about *strategies*, and when one becomes even more specific, about *targets*. Talk about strategies and targets thus provides an answer to the question, *How are you going to achieve this goal?* Thus, numerous strategies might be considered in pursuit of a single goal, and in turn, numerous targets might be considered in pursuit of a single strategy. No wonder, then, that talk about behavior change can be complex!

Table 4.3 is not intended to show the ideal weight-loss plan. Rather, it simply shows the range of potential topics for discussion in the consulting room, which move from the general to the specific. It is this movement which is important to note, not the precise definition of the terms *goals*, *strategy* and *target*. *Get more exercise* might be a goal for one person but a strategy towards another goal for someone else. The number of options for change increase as one becomes more specific.

Table 4.3 gives rise to a number of implications for practice. First, there is no point in talking about a target if the goal being pursued is not clear. Ideally, this goal should be chosen by the patient. Less obvious is how often we make the mistake of talking about a target without first checking whether another strategy might be more attractive to the patient, one which would give rise to an altogether different choice of targets. Using weight loss as the example again, there are so many options, admittedly some healthier than others, that it is worth checking which the patient would feel most confident in to begin with. Among the guidelines to emerge from this simple framework are the following:

Table 4.3   Goals, strategies and targets: from the general to the specific

Goal	→	Strategy	→	Target
Lose weight		1. Eat less fatty food		1. Cut out fried potatoes
				2. No red meat during the week
				3. No full-fat milk
		2. Start eating new food		1. Fruit once a day
		3. Replace certain foods		1. Baked potatoes or rice instead of chips
				2. Fish instead of meat at weekends
				3. Fruit instead of pudding 3/7 days
				4. Poached egg or beans on toast instead of bacon for breakfast
		4. Get more exercise		1. Walk to work whenever possible
				2. Arrange sport or dancing once a week
				3. Use the stairs instead of the lift.

- It is a good idea to get as far through this sequence as possible. *The more specific the target, the better*. Having said this, a premature leap to specificity can be dangerous.
- The patient is the expert in what is likely to work for him or her.
- There are often more options for change than patients realize. Opening up the discussion to examine alternatives and encouraging patients to choose those they feel most confident about is a useful activity (see Strategy 3 below).
- There is a lot of scope for providing information to patients about the wide range of options available and about the experiences of other patients.
- Levels of confidence to succeed will vary across and within an array of strategies and targets. Reassessing confidence can thus be used as an important guideline in selecting options (see Strategies 2 and 5).
- A patient's level of self-efficacy to achieve a specific goal will be determined by his or her confidence to achieve a wide array of smaller targets like those described in Table 4.3.

Resistance and building confidence

If a patient resists your efforts, consider which of the following might be the explanation:

- Are you focusing on building confidence when in fact the patient is not really convinced about the *importance* of the change under discussion? Consider a return to the task of exploring importance. You might even share this observation with the patient and allow him or her to be your guide.
- Are you overestimating the patient's level of confidence to succeed and unwittingly pushing him or her towards change? Back off! Consider reassessing confidence. Ask the patient how he or she really feels. Patients often simply cannot imagine coping without, say, a cigarette, a drink, or that special food in the fridge.
- Are you providing solutions rather than letting the patient discover them?
- Are you falling into the trap of talking about *single* solutions, when it is a little more complex for the patient?
- Are you looking at the 'wrong' target, or even the 'wrong' strategy for achieving change (see Table 4.3)? Clarify this with the patient.

A menu of strategies

A menu of strategies was constructed for exploring importance (see p. 77). A similar approach has been used here for deciding what strategy to use when helping patients with confidence issues. Choose a strategy that fits with the way the patient describes his or her lack of confidence. These strategies are not completely separate from one another. They are overlapping, being different ways to approach the subject of confidence building.

1. Do little more
2. Scaling questions
3. Brainstorm solutions
4. Past efforts: successes and failures
5. Reassess confidence

STRATEGY 1: DO LITTLE MORE

Most decisions to change do not take place in the consulting room. The patient does not necessarily need to set specific targets in conversation with you. It might be enough to simply raise the issue, mention the possibility of taking action, and leave it at that. If continuity of care is possible, this is often a very good starting point, much better, for example, than pushing too hard for change.

STRATEGY 2: SCALING QUESTIONS

This strategy is *linked to the numerical assessment of confidence* described in Chapter 3 (see p. 64). Once you are familiar with the process it will be easy to adapt it to non-numerical form, simply by asking questions. It is simply a way of opening the door to talk about strategies and targets. The patient, as you will see, does most of the thinking and talking while your role is to ask questions and help with clarifying the stumbling blocks to change.

How not to do it

Having obtained a numerical judgment from the patient about confidence to change, show no curiosity about how things could change. You could assume that you know what the patient should do, and proceed accordingly. Try some simple advice!

> *So you gave yourself a score of 3/10 for confidence to actually change your diet. What about cutting out those snacks between meals from now on?*

Towards good practice

Having conducted an assessment of how confident the person feels to make a particular change, you have been given a rating out of 10.

• You now have a platform for understanding exactly how the patient feels, and what might lead to successful change. Keep the pace of the discussion slow, and adopt a curious attitude. Your hope is that the answers lie within the patient.

- Ask either or both of the following questions, and then follow them on with other open questions or reflective listening statements.

1. 'Why so high?'

Ask why the patient scored a given number and not a lower number. *You said that you were fairly confident about your ability to change* [behavior]. *Why have you scored 4 and not 1?* The answers could provide important clues for what might work in the future. For example: *I am at 4 and not 1 because I know that if the situation is right, if I can keep away from friends who push me in the wrong direction, I can succeed.* This will allow you to respond with observations like: *So you've got the confidence to succeed if only you could organize your social life differently.* You can either pursue this in more detail, or keep the focus broad to begin with, by asking a question like: *What other reasons do you have for giving yourself a score of 4 and not 1?*

2. 'How can you go higher?'

You could also ask a quite different question, for example: *You gave yourself a score of 4. So you do have some confidence that you could succeed. How could you become more confident, so that your score goes up to 5 or 6?* or *What would help you to become more confident?* or *What stops you moving up from 4 to 5?* Note that one can ask about either *your score* or just *you*. The second method often feels like the better one.

STRATEGY 3: BRAINSTORM SOLUTIONS

Some patients, in some situations, apparently want to be told what to do. Certainly, if someone has an acute life-threatening condition, he or she will probably take your advice. In most behavior change consultations, however, patients probably prefer greater autonomy of decision making. If clinical judgment tells you that a patient really wants you to tell him or her what to do, then you should respond accordingly. However, most, we believe, will react against simple advice-giving.

The alternative to simple advice-giving is presented below in the form of a single strategy which can be learned quite quickly. In essence, rather than advising patients what to do, you encourage them to select targets and strategies for achieving them. Your expertise is used to enrich this process, not to overwhelm it. You construct a range of options with the patient, and then encourage him or her to choose the most appropriate one. You can suggest any number of options yourself, as long as you help the patient to choose that which is most suitable.

How do you help with action plans without telling patients what to do? How do you avoid falling into an advice-giving trap: the patient wants to know what to do, you offer a constructive suggestion, and then the patient tells you why this won't work? The problem with simple advice-giving is that it can restrict patients' sense of autonomy (see Chapter 2). Faced with this threat, they react against your advice. More information about the concept of reactance can be found in Miller & Rollnick (1991). Another problem with advice-giving is that it usually takes the form of a single, simple piece of advice. Surely, if it was that simple, the patient would have tried it before? You do not know the patient's circumstances as well as he or she does!

The strategy below is designed to maximize patient participation, while allowing you to use your knowledge and expertise to enhance this process, not to replace it. It is based upon identifying a range of possible options, and then helping the patient to select the most appropriate one.

How not to do it

If a patient says, *I don't know what to do about* ――, say: *Have you thought about* ――*?*. What usually happens is that the patient will tell you why your suggestion will not work. Then try another suggestion, and see what happens. However, you could try a more drastic approach: provide one single plan and force the patient to accept it while simultaneously expressing pessimism, for example: *There's only one way that's got any chance of success for you – if this doesn't work you'll never crack the problem.*

Towards good practice

This simple strategy is usually called *brainstorming*. However, the 'spirit' of this process is just as important as matters of technique. This should be conveyed to the patient from the outset.

1. Emphasize the principles

- *There is usually not one but many possible courses of action.*
- *I can tell you about what's worked for other people.*
- *You will be the best judge of what works for you.*
- *Let's go through some of the options together.*

2. Go through the options

Identify a number of options. Encourage the patient to come up with as many as possible. Use your expertise to suggest these options. Be careful about the patient becoming too passive. Try to avoid spending too much time evaluating the options. If the patient says, *Yes but, that won't work because ...*, say something like, *That's fine, let's not get too stuck on one idea, let's move on ... what else could you do?*

When presenting an option it can be useful to talk about what has worked for other patients. For example, *Some people in your situation have found it useful to ...* Another useful question is, *Are there any other ways that you know about that have worked for other people?*

Your attitude should be one of neutrality about the possibilities. It is up to the patient to decide. This is the next step.

3. Let the patient select the most suitable option

Questions like, *Which one suits you the best?* or *What makes the most sense to you?* will help the patient decide what to do. Your approach here is non-directive. Your task is to elicit and to understand how the patient really feels about what to do.

4. Convey optimism and willingness to re-examine

If the patient selects an option, let him or her know that if things don't work out there will be other options that might work. It is a matter of working out what best suits the individual.

Reminders

- This strategy can be used to select a goal, strategy or a target (see Table 4.3).
- Move from the general to the specific, not the other way around, i.e. from a goal, through strategies to targets.
- Help the patient set *small, achievable targets*, if at all possible.
- Establish a *realistic time scale*. Changing habits and establishing a new lifestyle takes time and is a gradual process. Some people enjoy dramatic all-or-nothing type changes but others cope better with gradual changes, one small step at a time. Choosing a day to begin the change can be important as well as choosing the pace of change. A good time scale is one which is slow enough to be manageable but fast enough to show some results so as to keep up the patient's motivation. Useful questions include: *One of the things you said you liked about drinking was the socializing – would there be any advantage in waiting until after Christmas before beginning to cut down?* or *You are a bit worried about your family's reaction if you start cooking the food with less fat – would you prefer to introduce this gradually to avoid a mutiny?* If you want to get it wrong, use clichés like: *No time like the present, In for a penny, in for a pound, If you can't do it now you never will, Might as well be hung for a sheep as for a lamb!*

- Is the patient really ready? Sometimes patients are not as ready as you thought, perhaps still being in the contemplation stage. This can account for their apparent resistance to selecting an option. Reassess readiness to change at any point. Be open about this with patients.
- Failing to make action plans does not mean that the consultation has failed. Do not push the patient too far. Time spent with you can often lead to action being taken independently at a later point.
- Clarify how you will both monitor progress.
- If behavior change does not take place, it is more helpful for both of you to see the plan, rather than the patient, as inadequate.
- Acknowledge patients' concerns, don't ignore them. Ask about these, if possible. Useful questions include: *You did say that you really enjoy the feeling of relaxation that you get from smoking. How much do you think you'll miss that?* or *Before we go on to plan how to change, are there any things that particularly concern you about the prospect of change …? What went wrong last time you tried and how will it be different this time? What takes people's confidence away?*

STRATEGY 4: PAST EFFORTS – SUCCESSES AND FAILURES

Our expectations of ourselves are frequently related to past experiences. We can learn what we are good at and what we find most difficult by looking back at previous attempts to change. This can be a good way of learning, a slightly more sophisticated form of *trial and error*. However, sometimes people allow their confidence to be undermined by what they see as repeated failures.

Helping someone to see the past as a valuable piece of information, to help plan a more successful future, is a skill. Patients with low self-esteem may be particularly likely to recount stories of their 'relapses' as evidence of their general worthlessness. 'Policing the past', as a colleague put it, can become a destructive part of clinic routine (N. C. H. Stott, personal communication). Here, the guilty patient feels obliged to explain failure to the well-meaning practitioner who routinely asks, 'How have you been getting on?', often merely as a device for starting the conversation about change.

How not to do it

Use words like *failure* and frame the question in terms of what the patient did wrong and is likely to do badly again, rather than in terms of a faulty plan or adverse circumstances which could be altered if another attempt was made.

You haven't been very successful in the past, have you? Perhaps we'd better take a long, hard look at what you did wrong last time and see if you can make a better go at it this time.

Towards good practice

Affirm the person's hard work and persistence in trying more than once. Courage and perseverance are important. Patients can be encouraged to give themselves credit for applying these qualities to the issue under discussion. Encourage them, too, to see themselves as competent, determined people who are potentially able to make changes but have not yet hit on a successful plan for doing so.

Ask about the person's most successful attempt to date. What made it different from any other attempts? Are any of these differences things that could, deliberately, be built into a new plan? Solution-focused therapists emphasize the value of encouraging people to talk about their strengths rather than their difficulties and to guide conversations towards 'solution talk' (Iveson & Ratner 1990).

Look for even transient evidence that change is possible. If someone feels it would be impossible to go half an hour or more without a cigarette, check if he or she has ever succeeded, even if he or she was coerced rather than chose such an action. Perhaps the person went on holiday by air or found him- or herself in a social situation where escaping for a cigarette was impossible for an hour or so. If someone finds it hard to imagine that he or she could refuse a drink offered by a friend, enquire if he or she has ever done so, for example when driving or on medication. How offended was the friend? Can anything from that situation be transferred over to the present?

If a patient acknowledges that he or she did change, briefly, but discounts this, saying, *Yes but it was dreadfully hard – it nearly killed me!*, he or she may be helped to reframe this as even more of a triumph: success in the face of almost overwhelming difficulty is worth acknowledging: *Looking back on it now you must be really impressed with yourself for coping with such a difficult situation!*

Keep the discussion of past experiences focused as much as possible on things that are, and are seen by the patient, as within his or her control. If a previous attempt failed because of unforeseen circumstances (*I was doing well going to the gym twice a week but then my husband lost his job and we had to sell the car* or *I was losing weight but then I fell pregnant and things were very difficult with the pregnancy and I really couldn't keep going with the diet plan then*), acknowledge that there were real difficulties and move on to look at things that the patient could plan for and take control over another time.

Warning!

It is easy to be over-positive about people's previous successes or too dismissive of unsuccessful attempts when trying to build confidence. This may lead to resistance in the form of a restatement of the patient's lack of confidence and a 'backing off' from the discussion. Look out for this and remain patient-centered. Chapter 5 contains more information on how to reduce resistance.

STRATEGY 5: REASSESS CONFIDENCE

The assessment of importance and confidence was pinpointed in Chapter 3 as something from which to launch a conversation about behavior change. In truth, it can be useful on an ongoing basis in the consultation, particularly when talking about confidence building. When one starts to talk about specific strategies and targets for confidence building, the levels of self-efficacy will vary across them. For example, someone wishing to change his or her diet might be more confident about eating more fruit, but less so about keeping away from chocolate.

To return to an assessment of levels of confidence can be very useful. This can be done formally, in numerical form, as described on p. 64, or it can be done informally, with a question like, *We have talked about change x and change y. Which of these do you feel more confident about succeeding with?* and later, *Why do you feel this way?* The obvious guiding principle is to encourage change which the patient is more likely to succeed with.

Case example: more talk about smoking

Nurse: *So you've tried to stop smoking lots of times before. How confident do you feel about having another go?*

Patient: *Not very.*

Nurse: *On a scale of 1 to 10, how confident do you feel? If 1 is 'not at all' and 10 is 'very' confident?* (Uses scaling questions)

Patient: *About 3 or 4.*

Nurse: *So, not very, but better than a 1 or a 2. How's that?* (Tries to elicit self-motivating statements)

Patient: *Well I tried cutting down gradually but that didn't work. I tried a 'quit smoking' group where they made us stop completely on a particular day. I once had a go with nicotine chewing gum. None of them worked in the long term but I did last 6 weeks once. That was with the quit group.*

Nurse: *What helped you to go so long that time?* (Reviews positives in previous attempt)

Patient: *I think it was better for me to stop completely. There was a nice woman in the group who I got on well with and we encouraged each other. It went wrong when I started seeing a man who smoked heavily and I had one ciggy one night and then just drifted back into it.*

Nurse: *So it sounds as if support from other people makes a big difference to you. It helps you to change* (Reviews positive experiences) *and when you spend a lot of time with someone who doesn't support you, you are more likely to slip back.* (Learns from previous failures) *It also sounds as if a definite quit date helps you?*

Patient: *Yes. I'm not very good at doing things on my own.* (Expresses low self-esteem in relation to behavior change in general)

Nurse: *There's nothing unusual about wanting support and that's why there are so many support groups set up. Shall we look at all the different ways you could get support this time if you decided to quit and see how you feel about them? Because of all the experience you've had of trying to change in the past you will be the best judge of what would work for you.* (Goes on to explore options and exchanges information as part of this process)

The nurse encourages the patient to draw on her previous experiences, not to make her remember her failures but to identify how much she has learned about herself and about stopping smoking. Her confidence will be built by seeing that if she does decide to change she can design her own action plan, incorporating the things she already knows can help her and working out how to cope with things that she can predict will be difficult.

It is important that the nurse remembers throughout that although the patient has agreed that it is important to change, she has not yet decided to do so. Adding the phrase *if you decided to quit* into the discussion about action plans avoids raising the resistance that might have been elicited by an implied assumption that the patient will change.

CONCLUSION

The skill required when talking to patients about the *why, how, what* and *when* of behavior change is not a matter of applying strategies *on* them, but of structuring a conversation in a useful way which encourages the patient to take as much of the lead as possible. Above all, it is about constructive listening and joint decision making. The strategies described in this chapter are merely guides to structuring this kind of consultation.

REFERENCES

Bandura A 1977 Towards a unifying theory of behavior change. Psychological Review 84:191–215

de Shazer S, Berg I, Lipchick E et al 1986 Brief therapy: a focused solution development. Family Process 25:207–222

Egan G 1994 The skilled helper: a problem management approach to helping. Brooks/Cole, Pacific Grove, CA

Iveson G, Ratner H 1990 Problem to solution. Brief Therapy Press, London

Miller W R 1983 Motivational interviewing with problem drinkers. Behavioural Psychotherapy 1:147–172

Miller W R, Rollnick S 1991 Motivational interviewing: preparing people to change addictive behavior. Guilford Press, New York

Orford J 1985 Excessive appetites: a psychological view of addictions. Wiley, New York

Rollnick S, Heather N, Bell A 1992 Negotiating behaviour change in medical settings: the development of brief motivational interviewing. Journal of Mental Health 1:25–37

Rollnick S, Butler C C, Stott N 1997 Helping smokers make decisions: the enhancement of brief intervention for general medical practice. Patient Education and Counseling 31:191–203

5

Exchange information and reduce resistance: two ongoing tasks

There are two tasks that a practitioner might need to perform at various stages throughout a consultation: exchanging information with the patient and responding constructively to resistance (Fig. 5.1). This final 'how to do it' chapter describes each of these in turn.

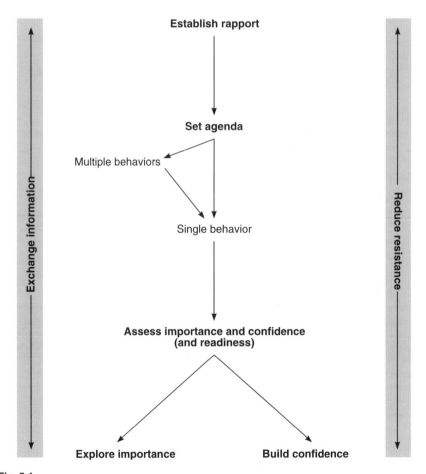

Fig. 5.1

Box 5.1 Useful Questions

Exchange information

1. *Would you like to know more about...?*
2. *How much do you already know about?*
3. *The test result is ... x, what do you make of this?*
4. *What happens to some people is – and –. What about you?*
5. *How do you see the connection between x and y?*
6. *Now that I have given you this information, how does it apply to you?*
7. *Take me through a **typical day** in your life, and tell me where your* [behavior] *fits in? ... So, on Monday, you woke up, how were you feeling? ... Then what did you do? ... You're going a bit fast for me! Can I take you back to when you left the house on Monday morning ... What happened then, and how did you feel?*

Reduce resistance
Asking the patient questions is not the best way to reduce resistance. However, it will be useful to ask **yourself** these questions instead! Remember, resistance is an observable behavior (e.g. denial, reluctance). It can be influenced by the goals you pursue and by the way in which you speak to the patient.

1. Have you undermined the patient's sense of personal freedom? Can you hand this control back?
2. Have you misjudged the patient's feelings about either readiness, importance or confidence? Have you jumped too far ahead of the patient on these dimensions? Are you focusing on the wrong dimension? Consider how this patient really does feel about change.
3. Are you meeting force with force? Are you being too confrontational? Can you do anything to come alongside the patient, or even change tack altogether?

TASK: EXCHANGE INFORMATION

An overweight, young woman is referred 'for dietary and fitness advice'. She sits down by your desk a little apprehensive and expectant. The overall task, as you both know, is to set her on the path to successful weight loss. You need to know some key things about her before you can imagine what might work for her. She is expecting you to give her information about diets and exercise. You expect that she has probably dieted before and has some knowledge and ideas about how to do it. You need to know how much she already knows and how accurate her existing information is. You want her to leave the consultation with all the accurate information she needs to make a success of a weight-loss program.

A middle-aged man has been diagnosed with liver disease. You need to discuss with him the importance of stopping drinking alcohol. You don't know whether he already realizes that he needs to think about his drinking. You don't know what part alcohol plays in his life and how much he would mind giving it up. You know a lot about strategies for giving up drinking and places he could get support and you would like to give him as much of this information as possible.

A large part of the practitioner's job is giving information to the patient. A large part of the patient's job is giving information to the practitioner.

Done badly, this task will make the patient a passive recipient of expert knowledge, disconnected from his or her context and concerns. Done well, it is a vehicle for true understanding and, it appears, a better outcome. For the practitioner, information exchange will be linked to specific medical or behavioral matters. For the patient it often also includes broader personal concerns. To deal with the former at the expense of the latter could be a serious mistake. Compliance can be enhanced by improving various aspects of the information exchange process. This is not just a 'technical matter' or an exercise in the exchange of facts, but something which involves the use of skillful listening, careful questioning and well-timed intervention. There are few parts of the consultation that do not involve the eliciting or providing of information.

Studies of communication reveal that the way in which practitioners exchange information can be strikingly one-sided and, at times, insensitive. For example, one study found that practitioners interrupted patients an average of 18 seconds into their initial description of the problem; in another, patients and practitioners did not agree on the main presenting problem in 50% of outpatient consultations (Starfield et al 1981).

Given its obvious importance, it is something of a surprise to notice that information exchange is seldom taught as a specific topic in its own right. It is difficult to find clear and teachable strategies that help practitioners to carry out this task. Rather, they are left to find their own ways of doing this. The purpose of this chapter is to bring together what we understand as the most effective and satisfying way to exchange information, in a form that can be learned and practiced. This is not only relevant to behavior change consultations. It also applies to other kinds of consultation, e.g. when breaking bad news, talking about diagnoses, and so on.

The lack of progress in developing such methods is not just a practical problem, but also a conceptual one. Information exchange has been too readily viewed as a one-sided process, hence the emphasis in both research and practice on either 'assessment' (getting information *from* the patient) or 'feedback' (giving information *to* the patient), both of which are activities derived mainly from the agenda of the practitioner. The education of medical and other students is usually guided by this kind of one-sided approach. As the strategies described below will reveal, the conceptual framework being used is explicitly a two-sided one, where the practitioner also encourages the patient to drive the discussion at certain points in the exchange process. Thus, the patient will not only be assessed and receive feedback, but will also express his or her information needs and be encouraged to arrive at a personal interpretation of the information received.

Conceived thus, information exchange is a skillful task which will benefit from further development work and from careful attention to the process of how best to improve competence among trainees. The details in this chapter are not the last word on this topic, but merely an attempt to open it up for further creative work by others.

The practical strategies below come from two sources: first, the study of communication and the patient-centered method; and second, motivational interviewing.

The patient-centered method

Research on communication reveals, as one might expect, that practitioners vary considerably in how they exchange information, and that outcome can be improved if information is clear and simple, and if practitioners negotiate and agree treatment goals in a cooperative manner (Becker 1985). Although these findings are obviously useful, much of the research on compliance is based on the notion that behavior change is best 'induced' by the expert-driven delivery of clear information, a view we explicitly reject (see Butler et al 1996).

Of more direct relevance has been the work on patient empowerment and the patient-centered method carried out by a number of North American research teams. Not all of this research focuses on information exchange, although a number of studies, reviewed by Stewart (1995), have looked explicitly at the process of history-taking. Four correlational studies, all of them in outpatient settings, reveal that during history-taking, activities like a full discussion of the problem, the asking of questions by the patient, providing information and giving emotional support, are all associated with better outcomes, such as the resolution of headaches and numerous other physical symptoms. Two randomized controlled trials found that practitioner training in history-taking improved levels of psychological distress in patients, and another two studies found that brief patient education (20 minutes) in how to ask questions not only improved participation but led to improved physical health such as control of blood pressure and blood glucose levels.

Of course, information exchange occurs not just during history-taking: a number of other studies of patient empowerment have involved the training of patients to be more assertive in other phases of the consultation. Thus, Innui et al (1976) found that giving patients greater control over what is talked about and encouraging them to seek personally relevant information can improve outcomes like control of blood pressure. Greenfield et al (1988) demonstrated that people with diabetes who were trained to be more involved in the consultation had better health outcomes than those who were not trained. Similarly, patients seen by health educators and coached to ask questions made better use of appointments over the following months (Roter 1977).

Finally, it is worth taking note of Silverman's (1997) observation of a feature of advice-giving which avoids being too personal and eliciting resistance: if the advice is couched in terms of information, i.e. in a broader, more neutral context, patients seem more likely to respond favorably.

In summary, there is clear evidence that if patients are more assertive during information exchange, outcomes can be improved. There is much less evidence that practitioners can be trained to improve their skills. There are clear correlations between elements of good-quality information exchange and patient outcome.

Motivational interviewing

A second source of innovation comes from the work of William R. Miller on motivational interviewing in the addictions field. He found a way of training counselors to encourage curiosity, question-asking and personal reflection among clients about the meaning of information provided to them. This process, it turns out, can have a powerful effect on people's decision-making. It appears that this is not just a matter of presenting appropriate information clearly to people, but of distinguishing between 'facts' and their interpretation. In these 'Drinker's Check-up' studies (see Miller & Sovereign 1989), the counselor provided the facts in a non-judgmental, neutral manner, and then encouraged the patient, through the use of simple open questions, to arrive at a personal interpretation of them. More detail about this process can be found in Miller et al (1988). The ideal outcome would be for the patient to say or think, *I see, I never thought about it like this before, I wonder if this means that …* Strategy 1, outlined below, is based on this aspect of motivational interviewing. It was refined further in the development of brief motivational interviewing (Rollnick et al 1992), where a clearly defined and documented information exchange strategy was taught to a group of general healthcare workers doing health promotion work with heavy drinkers in a general hospital (Heather et al 1996).

What emerges from these developments is a view of information exchange as part of a delicately balanced conversation. It does not need to be a sterile, expert-driven activity. From a conceptual viewpoint, we do not adhere to the view of information exchange as a practitioner-driven process either of eliciting facts from patients (assessment) or of providing them with information (feedback). In both such activities the patient will be driven along by the agenda of the practitioner, who will do most of the talking. Instead, we view the process in terms of the following circular *elicit–provide–elicit process*: first, patients are encouraged to describe their behavior, ask questions, indicate what they would most like to know, or disclose what they do and do not know about a particular topic (*elicit*). Unlike the more traditional approach, the practitioner is encouraged to adopt a curious and eliciting interviewing style during this phase, and the patient will do most of the talking. This is what is commonly called assessment. Second, the practitioner is active in conveying clear, non-judgmental information (*provide*) which, crucially, in the third phase, the patient is given an opportunity to absorb and reflect upon (*elicit*). We have distinguished between these three phases in order to develop teachable strategies. In reality, of course, they are usually interlinked, and might not follow a clear and logical sequence. This is not a problem. It is the spirit of information exchange that is most important.

What should happen if the practitioner has a very genuine desire to gather specific information from a patient close to the beginning of a consultation? How can one avoid firing, say, 20 closed questions at the patient? We are not saying that this kind of assessment has no place in a consultation. It can be useful, particularly when a reasonable rapport has been established, and it is done in a clear and logical manner. However, when working on the development of brief motivational interviewing we were interested to find a way of helping practitioners to gather information which was based more on a conversation, in a more patient-centered way. What emerged was the *Typical Day strategy* described below, in which the patient is simply encouraged to tell a story about a typical day. We were delighted with the way in which facts came tumbling out in this kind of account. It does take up to 6–10 minutes to use, and might therefore be beyond the scope of many consultations. If time is available, however, we recommend the use of this strategy as a viable alternative to asking the patient a large number of direct questions at the beginning of a consultation. Crucially, it helps to cement the rapport between the parties.

In summary, information exchange is an art as much as a technique or procedure. It is as much about maintaining rapport and having a conversation as it is about the exchange of facts. The two strategies outlined below are designed to help practitioners achieve these goals.

Fearful information: who wants it?

There is no shortage of fearful information in healthcare consultations, and usually it is the practitioner who decides that it will do the patient good to hear about it. Unfortunately, being concerned about risks and negative outcomes is not always a precipitant of change. We can all tell stories of patients who *increase* their risky behavior in the face of frightening information or experiences. Research in health psychology seems to bear this out (Schwartzer & Fuchs 1996). There are many other more positive motives for change, often little to do with health as such. If the patient asks about health risks and negative consequences, then of course it is appropriate to provide this. However, we should probably be careful of making a habit of providing frightening stories or facts. If we *are* going to develop a habit, the best is probably to routinely ask patients what they would like to know.

STRATEGY 1: GENERAL INFORMATION EXCHANGE
How not to do it

This is fairly straightforward. Adopt a patronizing tone of voice, make a decision that you think the patient needs information, and then 'wag your finger' at the patient; use the word 'you' as much as possible. Tell the patient exactly how to interpret the information, and throw in some direct persuasion as well, e.g. *Have you thought about how much damage smoking is doing to your lungs?* (without waiting for a reply). *If you don't stop smoking ... then you will find that your chest will get worse and worse over the next decade. I think you should seriously consider stopping before it is too late.* This kind of intervention is likely to generate resistance to change. The patient will feel cornered, and will not feel able to do anything but resist.

Towards good practice

The following principles are important:

- Does the patient want or need information? About what? How much does he or she already know? There is no point in providing irrelevant information or that which the patient does not want to receive. The best time to provide information is when the patient asks for it.
- Make a distinction, if at all possible, between factual information and the personal interpretation of it. You present the information and encourage the patient to interpret its meaning.
- When presenting information, present it in a neutral tone of voice, and avoid too much use of the word 'you'.

Consider the following sequence:

1. ELICIT readiness and interest

Ask the patient if he or she would like information, and about what? For example: *Would you like to know more about ——?* or *How much do you know about ——?* [then later] *Would you like to know how ——?* Do not rush this process. Take your time to understand what information, if any, the patient requires. If you get the feeling that the patient does not really want any information, back off and withdraw. In fact, don't appear too enthusiastic about the whole process!

2. PROVIDE feedback neutrally

Do this in a neutral manner, and try to avoid using the term 'you'. One way of achieving this is to refer to *other people*, and what happens to them. This is less threatening to the receiver and is thus more likely to be heard accurately. This knowledge about other people is also the true source of your expertise. *What happens to some people is that ... Other people find that...*

Follow the general principles of good information exchange:

- Use *language* you think the patient understands.

- Keep the *pacing* congruent with the person's uptake of the information; pause regularly to observe uptake and comprehension.
- Paint a general picture first, and then move into specifics as the patient directs you. To fill in too much detail can confuse people.

3. ELICIT the patient's interpretation, and follow it

Now is the time to use the word 'you'! The aim is to encourage the patient to make sense of the meaning of the information. *What do you make of this? I wonder how you have been affected by...?* Follow the patient's reaction for as long as you are able. This process of integrating information is what will help build motivation to change.

Taking home information

The principles described above also apply to information offered for taking home. Avoid 'distributing' information to patients. Assess their readiness to receive it first, and explain where in the literature they might locate the information most relevant to them. Invite them to return for further discussion.

STRATEGY 2: GATHERING INFORMATION – *A TYPICAL DAY*

This strategy emerged in the development of brief motivational interviewing (see Rollnick et al 1992), when we were looking for a way of conducting assessment in the form of a conversation led by the patient. The strategy is easily learned, provides the practitioner with a profusion of hard facts (usually the object of formal assessment) and also gives a clear idea about the relevant personal context of health behavior. Its usefulness extends beyond information exchange. It is ideal for establishing rapport. If focused on a particular behavior and its place in the person's life, it can also help to establish readiness to change.

This strategy involves simply asking the patient to take you through a typical day in his or her life. It is described here with reference to a particular behavior or problem, although this is obviously not essential. Having agreed to talk about a particular behavior or problem (e.g. diabetes), you can launch straight into this strategy. It can take as little as 3–5 minutes to use; the ideal time is about 6–8 minutes; too much longer and it can become tiresome for both parties. Of course, the strategy does not have to focus on a typical *day*. One can ask about a typical drinking or eating binge, a typical afternoon, or whatever.

The examination of a *typical* day, as opposed to, for example, a really difficult day, is somewhat arbitrary. One could use the latter approach, but our preference was for a focus on the normal, not the abnormal, as a device for establishing rapport and understanding the general context. Quite often, people tell you about the abnormal as part of this process. *It is a conversation, not an investigation.*

The *spirit* of this strategy is the most important: it is like asking the patient to paint a picture. Your role is simply to try to understand what is being painted. You might ask for a bit more detail here or there, but your task is simply to understand. The interviewing style is curious rather than investigative. This strategy is easy to practice with patients. We cannot recall its use causing discomfort. In broad outline, it takes the following form.

How not to do it!

Focus on a typical day, and fire a series of investigative questions at the patient, making sure that you understand the problem behavior in as much detail as possible. If you see an opening to be investigative and to pursue pathology, do so. Any other hypotheses you have should be investigated thoroughly!

> *When you say you **need** a drink after work, what exactly do you mean? When you say it calms you down are you generally an angry person? Why do you think that is? How did you learn to drink as a response to anger? Is this something your father used to do?*

Towards good practice

1. Introduce the task carefully

Sit back and relax! Ask the patient a question like: *Can you take me through a typical day in your life, so that I can understand in more detail what happens?* (Then, if you are talking about a particular behavior) *Then you can also tell me where your* [eating/smoking/drinking/ etc.] *fits in. Can you think of a recent typical day? Take me through this day from beginning to end. You got up…*

2. Follow the story

- Allow the patient to paint a picture with as little interruption as possible. Listen carefully. Simple open questions are usually all you need, for example: *What happened then? How did you feel? What exactly made you feel that way?*
- Avoid imposing any of your hypotheses, ideas or interesting questions on the story you are being told. Hold them back for a later time. This is the biggest mistake made when first using this strategy. Don't investigate problems!

- Watch the pacing. If it is a bit slow, speed things up: *Can you take us forward a bit more quickly? What happened when ...?* If it is a bit too fast, slow things down: *Hold on! You are going too fast. Take me back to ... What happened...?*
- If you are uncertain about details, and you are happy that you are being curious rather than investigative, then ask the patient to fill them in for you.
- You know you have got it right when you are doing 10–15% of the talking, the patient seems engaged in the process, and lots of interesting information about the person is emerging.

3. Review and summarize

Sometimes this is not necessary, and you can move on to another topic. If you do pause to take stock, a useful question is: *Is there anything else at all about this picture you have painted that you would like to tell me?* This is also a good opportunity to be honest with the patient about your reaction, and to provide affirmation wherever you can. Having listened so carefully to the patient, you will now be able to change the topic quite easily. Often this leads into the general information exchange strategy described above, introduced, for example by, *Is there anything about – that you would like to know?*

TASK: REDUCE RESISTANCE

Mrs Green's weight is a real problem. She says she would love to be slim. She is unresponsive, however, to any of your suggestions about healthy eating or physical activity. She does not accept that her weight is connected to her behavior in these areas; she says she hardly eats a thing and is always rushing around burning up energy. She is convinced the problem is 'glandular' or genetic in some way. You don't know how to help when she won't accept your suggestions.

Her husband, on the other hand, agrees with you that it would be good for him to be more active. However, for every good idea you have he has a reason why he cannot do it. He hates ball games, he can't afford to join a gym, walking to and from work is too dangerous in his neighborhood with the late shifts he does and the pool isn't open at hours that suit him.

Some patients seem to resist your best efforts to help them. You think you are making good progress and then it all gets difficult again.

The discussion that follows leans unashamedly on motivational interviewing, with the goal of identifying some of the most useful ideas that can be applied to brief consultations. The three practical strategies to follow are simply examples of the ways in which practitioners can respond to resistance. It is an area with rich potential for further development and research. We have focused on generally applicable strategies, and stopped short of looking at a range of problem consultations which could clearly benefit from further development work, for example, in talk about chronic pain or chronic fatigue syndrome, where the levels of resistance can be very high. Other useful ideas can be found in the work of Egan (1994), who captures much of what is said in this chapter by noting, 'Effective helpers neither court reluctance or resistance nor are surprised by it' (p. 151).

What is it?

It is hard to imagine a behavior change consultation which is not visited by resistance. It can be felt almost like an electrical current, and arises when there is tension or disagreement about behavior change. Since this can arise at any point in the consultation, it requires continual watchfulness. Its equivalent in dancing is the paying of attention to keeping yourself and your partner from stepping on each other's toes. Maintaining a lightness of touch is essential.

The forms of resistance that emerge will vary across consultations and contexts. Sometimes it takes the form of quiet reluctance in the patient, at other times as outright denial. Our impression is that in most healthcare settings it manifests in quiet reluctance, although scrutiny of talk about chronic fatigue syndrome reveals that it approaches the kind of overt conflict typically encountered in the addictions field. Here, there is a tradition in some treatment centers for headstrong clients, embattled by years of conflict over their addiction, to meet their match: they are confronted by stridently directive counselors with 'the problem', and react with predictable defensiveness (resistance). One account of this process even referred to it as giving the client an 'emotional haircut' (Yablonsky 1989). Although healthcare practitioners, in our experience, seldom work in this way with patients, they can become battle-weary from too many frustrating encounters with difficult patients. Attitudes can harden and are expressed by statements like, 'These patients are all the same. They simply don't want to look after themselves'. The danger here is that legitimate assessments about some patients harden into downright prejudice.

In many healthcare consultations there appears to be less outright conflict, perhaps because time is shorter and patients do not have such a history of conflict with their carers. Practitioners, for their part, sometimes tread a skillful path in order to avoid conflict (Butler et al 1998). Certainly, practitioners know well that one way to avoid resistance is not to raise the subject of behavior change in the first place. This delicate management of resistance is well illustrated in the account of Silverman (1997) who describes quiet reluctance (e.g. 'uhmm') from patients more commonly than outright rejection. The need to 'save face' by both parties might be one explanation for this (Silverman 1997). We recently had the opportunity to listen to recordings of consultations about coughs, colds and sore throats, where discomfort for doctors about whether or not to prescribe antibiotics is well documented in the literature (Bradley 1992). We found very little resistance, and reached the conclusion that both parties conduct a delicate dance around the subject of antibiotics. Patients are seldom asked outright whether they want this medication, and doctors often avoid mentioning the word. Yet both parties know that it is a central issue. In other words, the subject of resistance is not new to healthcare practitioners and patients: many are artful managers of tension in talk about change!

A description of various forms of resistance can be found in Chamberlain et al (1984): *arguing* can take the form of challenging, discounting and outright hostility; *denying* can manifest in blaming, disagreeing, excusing, claiming impunity, minimizing, pessimism and reluctance; two other categories are *interrupting* and *ignoring*, which include behaviours like inattention, non-answer and sidetracking (see also Miller & Rollnick 1991).

What causes resistance?

Resistance can arise when the patient brings conflict into the consulting room, when the practitioner elicits it, or as a result of a combination of the two.

The patient can be in a state of internal conflict about change in which different voices in the mind are pressing for different outcomes: *I want to but it's so difficult ...; I may as well just carry on ... If I could only try one more time ...* The stronger and more conflicting the voices, the more likely it is that resistance will arise. If the person is in conflict with others as well, it can be even more pronounced: *She always nags me about my diet, but she's the one who makes the food in the first place. How can I help it?* And sometimes the person might not be in a state of conflict, but one of learned helplessness about lifestyle change. For example, some patients with chronic conditions like diabetes develop an almost habitual feeling of reluctance to change their lifestyles, and the routine check-up is characterized by reluctance from the patient and frustration for the practitioner. The more someone feels obliged to attend an appointment, the more likely it is that the consultation will be dogged by resistance.

Whatever the personal source of resistance for the patient, *he or she will be particularly sensitive to the way he or she is spoken to.* Problems usually arise in the consultation when, wittingly or unwittingly, the practitioner, wanting to encourage change, elicits from the patient a voice for no change: *Have you thought about controlling your diet?* The temperature is raised, and the stage is set for the emergence of resistance. *Yes, but...*

In some circumstances resistance can arise in the complete absence of conflict in the patient, when it is the practitioner who is concerned about change. For example, a heavy drinker with no associated medical problems and who has never thought about alcohol use as a problem, is at the receiving end of a health promotion effort intended to minimize future complications. If the practitioner implies that alcohol use is a problem, resistance is a predictable outcome. More common, we suspect, is where the origin of resistance is not as extreme as in this example, and there is an interaction between the conflict experienced by the patient and the motives and consulting behavior of the practitioner. Thus, whatever its origins, resistance cannot be defined outwith this *interpersonal* context. The practitioner has the potential to lower or raise the level of resistance.

Dealing with resistance

It is unrealistic to view resistance as a sign of failure in the consultation, something which is abnormal and should be eliminated from the discussion at all costs. Some therapists even say that with good rapport, resistance provides the kind of energy that generates change. However, in most time-limited healthcare consultations it is a nuisance. Hence our view that, on an ongoing basis, practitioners should look out for resistance and move towards reducing it. This is not just a matter of what you say, or what strategy you use, but how you say it, and being in a flexible state of mind in which you *roll with resistance* (Miller & Rollnick 1991) and avoid argument.

Three traps: three strategies

Three traps have been isolated for particular attention, each giving rise to a strategy for avoiding it which is described below. Fall into any of these traps and resistance will be a likely outcome.

1. Take control away We all know some patients who are very compliant and like to be told what to do. Most, however, do not respond well to this. Strategy 1 below (*Emphasize personal choice and control*) illustrates how one can avoid this pitfall in a consultation.

2. Misjudge importance, confidence or readiness This is a very common trap to fall into. For example, one can focus prematurely on change when the patient is not ready for this, or one could focus on importance when the patient is actually more concerned about confidence matters. Strategy 2 below (*Reassess readiness, importance and confidence*) involves re-examining the patient's feelings about these issues, to make sure that one remains aligned to his or her needs.

3. Meet force with force Whatever the topic of conversation is, whoever the patient is, confronting resistance with force will make matters worse. A consultation is not like a wrestling contest! Of all the strategies described below, this is the most skillful to execute. However, use of Strategy 3 below (*Back off and come alongside the patient*) will demonstrate that the rewards are liberating.

Awareness of strategies for dealing with resistance should not overshadow the most important guideline: watch, look and listen. If you meet resistance, change tack. Simply being aware of it, and not making it worse, often leads quite directly into the use of strategies outlined below, sometimes quite unconsciously. This is certainly not just a technical matter of using this or that strategy, but of being in a watchful and flexible frame of mind, and remembering that you do not have to feel responsible for providing a counter-argument. Resistance is often a signal to you to change gear and to repair damaged rapport, usually by coming alongside patients and talking in a way more in sympathy with their feelings and attitudes. Be watchful for the patient who is in verbal accord with you, but whose body language demonstrates obvious resistance.

STRATEGY 1: EMPHASIZE PERSONAL CHOICE AND CONTROL

If a person is struggling to maintain some sense of control over his or her life, it does not take much to threaten this sense of stability. All one needs is a confrontation with a practitioner, and resistance to change will emerge. It does not take much to fall into the trap of undermining the personal autonomy of the patient. Statements like *You should do ...* or *The biggest problem you have is ...* are likely to have this effect, because they restrict the person's sense of freedom and will elicit resistance in the form of reassertion of autonomy (see Miller & Rollnick 1991). Every parent knows this problem: if you say to a young child, *You are dirty and you should go and wash now*, the almost instinctive reaction will be a form of resistance, which has more to do with personal autonomy being undermined than with the content of your statement. The content, e.g. a response from the child like, *But I'm not dirty*, merely provides the stage on which the battle for autonomy is played out.

Practitioners, even when giving advice, appear to be well aware of these subtleties and apparently adjust their message accordingly, hence the discovery by Silverman (1997) that they make their advice ambiguous so as to avoid becoming too personal: they present their advice in neutral terms, as if it is information. Another viable option to avoid threatening autonomy is to make this explicit. A simple phrase added on to a piece of advice can make all the difference: *I think that you should stop smoking now, but it's really up to you*. This might well avoid eliciting resistance. Leave out the second half, and you could be in trouble.

It is also not merely a matter of *what* is being said, but *how* it is being said. The practitioner's attitude and the atmosphere of the consultation will contribute to the patient's reaction. The same words used in two different atmospheres will have quite different effects.

A useful way of capturing the subtleties of this trap is to note that a confrontational interviewing style is likely to undermine autonomy and elicit resistance. This observation, which provided the starting point for motivational interviewing (see Miller 1983), has been borne out in a number of studies which demonstrate that what happens in the consulting room affects patient outcome (Chamberlain et al 1984, Miller & Sovereign 1989). One study, for example, among help-seeking problem drinkers found that the number of confrontational statements made by counselors correlated with the amounts that patients drank at follow-up (Miller et al 1993). The need to avoid confrontational interviewing provides the rationale for basing this method on essential listening skills, which are the antithesis of confrontational interviewing, and for the assertion that the spirit of this method is more important than any strategy being employed (see p. 32). The examples below illustrate this process of handing control back to the patient.

How not to do it

Look out for a patient who seems reluctant to consider change, who is struggling to maintain control over his life, and suggest firmly that you think he should change. Ignore any resistance, even it is a quiet form of reluctance, and proceed with advice-giving in discharge of your duty.

Towards good practice

Many situations serve to undermine this sense of autonomy, and are often associated with resistance to change. Handing this back to the patient can be done in many ways. Indeed, the assessment of readiness, importance and confidence (Strategy 2, below) is one way of encouraging patients to say exactly how they feel about change. So too, going through an agenda-setting exercise (Chapter 3) has this goal as its explicit purpose.

If the patient is to be an active decision maker, he or she must feel in control of choices that are made. These choices are about both what is talked about in the consultation, and what the patient should do outside the consulting room.

Diabetes, diet and agenda setting

The patient attends a clinic for a routine check-up:

Practitioner: [After going through medical matters and feeding back the result of a blood test]. *And how's your food intake going?*

Patient: *OK*

Practitioner: *How do you feel it is going?* (Practitioner tries again)

Patient: *Well, I try, but sometimes I break the rules, as you know.*

Practitioner: *I guessed that.*

Patient: *You see, it's been so busy, it's hard to always think about all this.*

Practitioner: *I can imagine.* (Practitioner decides to shift focus and start again with agenda setting) *Can we stand back from this for a moment, and understand how you feel about the meeting today? What would you like to talk about today? We could talk about eating, exercise, your medication or any of the usual things. But how do you feel? Perhaps there's something more pressing for you today that we could talk about?* (See Chapter 3 for an outline of this strategy)

Patient: *Well, one thing I do know is that…*

This next example is a brief version of the same strategy, handing control back to the patient:

Dietary advice

Practitioner: *You say you would like some dietary advice. Have I ever shown you this record sheet? The idea is that you keep a record on a daily basis for the next week.*

Patient: *No, but I've tried that sort of thing once before. It was just hopeless.* (Resistance)

Practitioner: *I understand. I wonder what you think will be most helpful to you?*

Patient: *Well, what I need to do is to be able to…*

In this next example, the patient's sense of control over a heart attack is delicately balanced, and unwittingly undermined by the practitioner's action talk. Once again, the practitioner tries to give the patient control over what is talked about in the consultation.

Exercise, the fear of a heart attack and a shift to information exchange

Practitioner: [Aiming to build confidence about behavior change] *So these exercises are specially designed to help someone like you who has had a heart attack, to help you slowly get back on your feet again.*

Patient: *OK, thanks.* (Little conviction)

Practitioner: *You can do them once a day to start off with, perhaps soon after you get up in the morning.*

Patient: *uhmmm.* (Possible resistance)

Practitioner: [Wondering whether the above apparent agreement is in fact resistance] *There's something worrying you about doing that.*

Patient: *Well how do I know that I won't have another heart attack?*

Practitioner: *You think, perhaps, that too much exercise might make things worse.*

Patient: *Well, that's right, couldn't it?*

Practitioner: [Realizes that there is something else of greater concern to the patient] *Do you think we should chat for a minute or two about the risk and that sort of thing?* (Shifting focus to information exchange)

Patient: *Well you can't help wondering when its going to happen again.*

Practitioner: *How do **you** understand what is happening to your heart?* (First phase of information exchange, i.e. elicit the patient's understanding).

In this example the practitioner made a decision to focus on confidence building, but the patient was more concerned about something else. The control over what was to be discussed was not given to the patient to begin with. The observation of resistance provided the basis for the practitioner's decision making in the consultation, to shift focus from a confidence building strategy to an information exchange strategy – one which in this case assumed less readiness to change. By understanding the source of this resistance, (*'There's something worrying you about doing that'*) the practitioner was able to find a task (information exchange) which was congruent with the needs of the patient, and gave her greater control over what was talked about and any decision making about behavior change.

STRATEGY 2: REASSESS READINESS, IMPORTANCE OR CONFIDENCE

A common cause of resistance is when the practitioner falls into the trap of overestimating or misjudging readiness, importance or confidence. Most often, this results in premature action talk. If readiness is seen as a continuum, and the patient is at the not-ready end, practitioner talk which assumes that the patient either is or should be at the ready end (action talk) will elicit resistance. Seen in this light, resistance is a measure of the extent to which the practitioner has jumped ahead of the patient (Rollnick et al 1993). The obvious practical implication is that a shift in the practitioner's strategy is necessary to ensure congruence with the patient's state of readiness. The same overestimation mistake can be made when the talk is about either the importance of change or the confidence to achieve it. For example, a practitioner establishes that a smoker would very much like to give up (i.e. importance is high), but the smoker is concerned about achieving this (confidence is low). The practitioner makes the mistake of assuming that this confidence should be higher and more amenable to shifting than it really is, and that a few bits of simple advice will suffice. Some suggestions are offered. The outcome is resistance.

This discussion has assumed that the patient would like to talk about behavior change. However, a more dramatic, yet very common, example of overestimation is to focus on behavior change when the patient is more concerned about something else. Thus the exercise specialist talks about exercise when a patient in cardiac rehabilitation is feeling depressed and fearful about having another episode of myocardial ischemia; or the patient attending a diabetes clinic is in a hurry to get to the shops, and does not wish to talk about diet.

A practitioner can also *misjudge* (rather than overestimate) a patient's feelings, by focusing on confidence instead of importance, or vice versa. This is a common mistake to make. Might this be the problem with the husband of the woman described above, who is actually not convinced about the importance of change, while the discussion focuses on confidence? People often come into action-orientated clinics and slip into talk about practical measures to improve confidence to change. Healthcare practitioners are trained to do things to people, and to solve problems. Nothing is easier than providing a few simple bits of advice!

How not to do it

Assume that it does not matter how ready the patient is, or what his or her feelings are about importance or confidence. Act accordingly.

Towards good practice

If you have made the mistake of either overestimating one of these qualities or focusing on the wrong one, the most obvious response to the resistance that can arise is to re-evaluate the direction you are taking. This can be done explicitly, by asking the patient to tell you how he or she really feels, particularly about the distinction between importance and confidence. This can be achieved in a few minutes.

This reassessment does not necessarily have to be done in an explicit manner, but can be achieved simply by sharing with the patient your confusion about what exactly his or her concerns are. Here is an example of what one might say to the husband cited above on page 114.

Practitioner: *How do you feel about being more active?*

Patient: *I'd like to, yes.*

Practitioner: *Have you thought about what kind of activity suits you?*

Patient: *It's not so easy for me. I hate sports and competition; I never did like that sort of thing.*

Practitioner: *What about walking?* (Practitioner tries to focus on confidence building)

Patient: *It's not safe where I live. I come off my shift late at night and it's madness out there … These kids are wild, like they just don't care about anyone.*

Practitioner: *And a gym?* (Is the practitioner focusing on confidence instead of importance?)

Patient: *I can't afford that sort of thing.*

Practitioner: (Does the patient feel that exercise is not really that important to him? A decision is made to see whether the talk about confidence is a mistake. This could be done explicitly, by asking the patient to rate importance and confidence on a scale from 1 to 10, but on this occasion, the shifting of gear in the face of resistance is done more subtly) *I'm not sure what to think. Perhaps you are feeling that there's no easy solution here, and that there are other things that are more important to you right now than getting more exercise.*

Patient: *Well, you know what I mean, sometimes one just has to put up with what life throws at you, like I've got a lot going on at the moment and who knows how I can get more exercise.*

Practitioner: *It's hard to see how to fit it all in.*

Patient: *That's right, I'm not a perfect machine, I'm more like a reliable old car…*

Practitioner: *Maybe now's not the time for a tune up.*

Patient: *Who knows, I don't really know what to do.*

STRATEGY 3: BACK OFF AND COME ALONGSIDE THE PATIENT

This strategy is designed to counter the trap of meeting force with force. It captures this heart of motivational interviewing, i.e. responding to resistance by keeping in a state of mind in which one does not 'take the bait' or meet force with force, but comes alongside the patient. The technique of making reflective listening statements is a direct way of achieving this.

How not to do it

Attack or defend. Argue forcefully for change, and meet arguments with yet more counter-arguments. You will both feel tired and frustrated.

Towards good practice

The spirit

Avoiding argument is not just a passive process in which one sits back in a defensive posture and uses reflective listening until the fire dies down, but one in which the practitioner tries to come alongside the patient and understand how he or she is feeling. If successful, the resistance will usually subside, and the discussion can move in a different direction.

The technique

Reflective listening involves making statements designed to show that you understand the meaning of what the person is saying (see Miller & Rollnick 1991). The effect of using such statements, as opposed to questions, is to encourage the patient to continue talking and expressing his or her views and feelings. Figure 2.4 in Chapter 2 can be a useful aid for understanding this process. The reflective statements can take a variety of forms: repeating exactly what the person has said, rephrasing it in different words; or adding new meaning to that expressed by the patient. These statements often begin with words like, *So you ...*, *You feel ...*, *Its ...* and *You...*

A common example

In this example, the entire sequence is characterized by the use of reflective listening. We are not implying that questions are not useful, but simply want to illustrate how far one can go with reflective listening. In reality, one might use a fair proportion of questions and summary statements. The goal of coming alongside the patient is what matters.

Exercise or diet?

Practitioner: *I wonder what would suit you best, to look at your eating or to think about taking more exercise?*

Patient: *I get as much exercise as I want, and every time I try to diet I end up eating the fried foods that the kids get.* (Resistance)

Practitioner: *You don't want to try something that's not going to work.* (A reflective listening statement which aligns practitioner with patient, and does not increase the resistance)

Patient: *That's right, if I could do something with the diet, I would.*

Practitioner: *You can't see a way forward on this one at the moment.* (Another reflection)

Patient: *But what if I carry on the way I am?*

A serious bush fire!

Occasionally people come into the consulting room feeling very cross. The potential for a serious inflammation is obvious. This next example illustrates how coming alongside the person and using reflective listening can build rapport and avoid serious conflict. It is a verbatim transcript of a simulated encounter between Dr Terri Moyers and a professional actor playing the role of someone obliged to see a counselor by a court of law (Miller et al 1998). Neither party was prepared beforehand about how the consultation would proceed. Although the context is outside of healthcare, its relevance to the occasional difficult consultation in healthcare settings is striking.

Dr Moyers: *Well Jim, I'm glad you're here. I'm kind of surprised to see you're coming back today.*

Client: *Well, I tell you one thing. I sat out the front here for about an hour before I came in and I was just about that close to cranking that pick-up up and heading back home. I'll let you know just like I told Rich, I'm not real happy about being here. I hope you understand that.*

Dr Moyers: *I'm hearing you loud and clear that being here is not something that is a high priority for you.*

Client: [Chuckling] *I'm looking at you and you've got blonde hair. I haven't had a lot of luck with blonde hair in the last couple of weeks.*

Dr Moyers: *Is that right? Well tell me a little bit more about that.*

Client: *Well, I got assigned a probation officer and she's a blonde-haired girl and I think she's out to destroy me totally.* (Visibly upset) *She's talking about me getting a lot of jail time, and this big fine and everything she's going to do if I don't do certain things. I just kind of think maybe you're going to do the same thing to me.*

Dr Moyers: *So it seems to you like I might try to push you around and make you do a whole bunch of things that you don't want to do.*

Client: *Yes. I'm about up to here with this kind of stuff. I hope you know that. It probably isn't your fault but I just kind of – the way things have been going you know.*

Dr Moyers: *You're pretty fed up.*

Client: *I am. My daughter, you know, she won't let me see the kids.*

They talk for 1–2 minutes about this. Then the client returns to his anger about being obliged to attend counseling.

Client: *... I've got about 3 more years to go before I retire so a lot of what I'm doing here, why I'm coming here is so that I can maybe save my driver's licence, I won't lose my job, I won't lose my house. It's not because I want to do any of this crap* [he means the counseling].

Dr Moyers: *You're not here because you think you have a problem. You're here because they sent you here.*

Client: *Yes, the court sent me here.*

Dr Moyers: *That's the only reason you're here.*

Client: *Yes. I'll be honest with you. No need in my lying to you unless you go down and tell the court that I'm not motivated to be here. I don't like any of this. I'll be honest with you. It's taken a lot of time that I don't have. It's taken a lot of money that I don't have, for the court and the fines and all that stuff and on top of that I have to pay my lawyer $1000 which I don't have, to represent me. I guess he's probably one of the reasons I'm here today because he and I drink together. I've known this guy ever since he got out of law school. He's a good friend of mine. I say* [to him] *why have I got to go up there? I'm paying you $1000 to represent me and now I've got to go over and go through this evaluation and all that. Now that doesn't make sense and he's saying you've got a drinking problem. Hell, you know I've had to take him home a lot of times. I've been the one standing and he's been passed out and couldn't walk. This just doesn't make sense. None of this makes sense.*

Dr Moyers: *So it's confusing to you why your drinking should cause a problem or everybody should be talking about that when you look around and you see that other people drink more than you do.*

Client: *Well at this point in my life. It would be different now. I mean*

10 years ago I probably would have taken my medicine without being too cranky about it but let me tell you something. I've changed an awful lot in 10 years. I used to be a rounder, I used to fight, I used to rodeo. I used to drink a lot. I made a living hauling rodeo stock and everything and now I've settled down the last 8/10 years. I've got my good job, I'm driving short-distance hauls. I drink a little bit but I work hard. It's nothing for me to sit down and drink a six-pack of beer and still be able to function. I'm not like one of them bums you see laying down there by the bus depot on the lawn selling his blood and stealing hub caps. I've never stole anything and I've worked every day since I've got a social security card.

Dr Moyers: *So it's kind of the same thing as you were saying before, which is that it feels like everybody is looking at your drinking but it's not as bad as everybody thinks it is.*

Client: *You might say that. I don't know that it's true but you might say that.*

In this interview Dr Moyers managed to avoid falling into the first and third traps described above. She was careful not to take control away from the client and to avoid meeting force with force. She did this by trying to come alongside the patient, to understand things from his perspective. She used mainly reflective listening statements to achieve this goal. She avoided asking too many questions because they can sometimes have the effect of passing control over what is talked about back to the practitioner.

Concluding note

We have covered three traps in this discussion of resistance. There are undoubtedly others that the practitioner can fall into which lead to resistance. These are merely the most commonly occurring ones that we have come across. For example, what if the patient wants more or less direction than the practitioner is offering? This is one of the most puzzling and challenging aspects of behavior change consultations which is discussed in more detail in Chapter 8. A mismatch of this kind is likely to lead to resistance. Clearly, more work needs to be done on this issue.

The challenge for practitioners is first to develop an awareness of resistance and then to practice being flexible in response to it, to maintain a lightness of touch which allows them to avoid meeting force with counter-argument.

Resistance is a key to successful treatment if you can recognize it for what it is: an opportunity. In expressing resistance, the client is probably rehearsing a script that has been played out many times before. There is an expected role for you to play –

one that has been acted out by others in the past. Your lines are predictable. If you speak these same lines, as others have done, the script will come to the same conclusion as before. But you can rewrite your own role ... Resistance lies at the heart of the interplay. It arises from the motives and struggles of the actors. It foreshadows certain ends to which the play may or may not lead. The true art of therapy is tested in the recognition and handling of resistance. It is on this stage that the drama of change unfolds. *(Miller & Rollnick, 1991 p. 111–112)*

REFERENCES

Becker M H 1985 Patient adherence to prescribed therapies. Medical Care 23:539–555

Bradley C P 1992 Uncomfortable prescribing decisions: a critical incident study. British Medical Journal 304:294–296

Butler C C, Rollnick S, Stott N C H 1996 The practitioner, the patient and resistance to change: recent ideas on compliance. Canadian Medical Association Journal 154:1357–1362

Butler C C, Rollnick S, Pill R, Maggs-Rapport F, Stott N 1998 Understanding the culture of prescribing: a qualitative study of general practitioners' and patients' perceptions of antibiotics for sore throats. British Medical Journal 317:637–642

Chamberlain P, Patterson G, Reid J, Kavanagh K, Forgatch M 1984 Observation of client resistance. Behavior Therapy 15:144–155

Egan G 1994 The skilled helper: a problem management approach to helping. Brooks/Cole, Pacific Grove, CA

Greenfield S, Kaplan S H, Ware J E, Yano E M, Frank H J 1988 Patients' participation in medical care: effects on blood sugar control and quality of life in diabetes. Journal of General Internal Medicine 3:448–457

Heather N, Rollnick S, Bell A, Richmond R 1996 Effects of brief counselling among male heavy drinkers identified on general hospital wards. Drug and Alcohol Review 15:29–38

Innui T S, Yourtree E L, Williamson J 1976 Improved outcomes in hypertension after physician tutorials. Internal Medicine 84:646–651

Miller W R 1983 Motivational interviewing with problem drinkers. Behavioral Psychotherapy 1:147–172

Miller W R, Rollnick S 1991 Motivational interviewing: preparing people to change addictive behavior. Guilford Press, New York

Miller W R, Sovereign R 1989 The check-up: a model for early intervention in addictive behaviors. In Loberg T, Miller W R, Nathan P E, Marlatt G A (eds) Addictive behaviors: prevention and early intervention. Swets & Zeitlinger, Amsterdam

Miller W, Sovereign G, Krege B 1988 Motivational interviewing with problem drinkers: II. The drinker's check-up as a preventative intervention. Behavioral Psychotherapy 16:251–268

Miller W, Benefield R, Tonigan S 1993 Enhancing motivation for change in problem drinking: a controlled comparison of two therapist styles. Journal of Consulting and Clinical Psychology 61:455–461

Miller W R, Rollnick S, Moyers T 1998 Motivational interviewing: professional training videotape series. University of New Mexico: Albuquerque

Rollnick S, Heather N, Bell A 1992 Negotiating behaviour change in medical settings: the development of brief motivational interviewing. Journal of Mental Health 1:25–37

Rollnick S R, Kinnersley P, Stott N 1993 Methods of helping patients with behaviour change. British Medical Journal 307:188–190

Roter D L 1977 Patient participation in the patient provider interaction: the effects of question asking on the quality of interaction, satisfaction, compliance. Health Education Monograph 5:281–315

Schwarzer R, Fuchs R 1996 Self-efficacy and health behaviours. In: Conner M, Norman P (eds) Predicting health behaviour: research and practice with social cognition models. Open University Press, Buckingham

Silverman D 1997 Discourses in counselling: HIV counselling as social interaction. Sage: London

Starfield B, Wray C, Hess K et al 1981 The influence of patient–practitioner agreement on outcome of care. American Journal of Public Health 71:127–131

Stewart M 1995 Effective physician–patient communication and health outcomes: a review. Canadian Medical Association Journal 152:1423–1433

Yablonsky L 1989 The therapeutic community: a successful approach for treating substance abusers. Gardner Press, New York

PART III

Application

6

Common clinical encounters

Part II of this book contains a collection of strategies linked to a series of common tasks in behavior change consultations. The aim of this chapter is to illustrate how these can be used in different situations. Because of the striking uniformity in talk about behavior change, these strategies should be widely applicable. The same topics of conversation arise again and again. Yet there is also remarkable diversity, where each encounter is a unique conversation, in which a practitioner must adapt the strategy to suit the situation. The clinical scenarios below are not intended to be models of good practice, but illustrations of how a practitioner can use the toolbox in a range of situations. The first section of this chapter provides some general guidelines for using the toolbox, while the second contains examples of application in a range of settings.

SOME GUIDELINES

Spirit and technique

To become bogged down in matters of technique and strategy can lead one away from the more important spirit of these consultations about behavior change. The variety of techniques that could be used is almost endless, but as noted in Chapter 2 (p. 32), the spirit is more enduring. Some practitioners will want more structure to guide their work than others.

The metaphor of a toolbox has its limitations. In truth, while the tasks we have identified are clearly defined, the strategies are not really like tools in a toolbox, because one will always want to adapt and refine them to suit the individual.

Practice

A 3- to 5-minute consultation in an emergency room with an alcohol user will be different from a 20-minute review of multiple behaviors with a patient who has chronic diabetes. This method covers a broad area. You need to ask, 'How does it fit into my context?'. Some parts will be useful, others less so or even irrelevant. As an individual practitioner, trying things out with patients will do them no harm, because of the emphasis placed upon active, empathic listening in the method. You will soon learn what suits your patients, your context and your consulting style.

Consider a menu

We have structured the method described in Part II around a set of tasks which follow a roughly sequential order in a consultation. One does not necessarily need to be restricted by this structure. One useful starting point is simply to construct a menu of strategies which you consider important for application in your everyday work. We have observed groups of colleagues readily reaching consensus about what tasks match their needs, and what a provisional menu of strategies might look like. Some menus might have a stronger sequential order than others. The outcome is freedom for practitioners to choose a strategy at any given moment in the consultation.

Stop! Do you know what you are doing?

This is a useful general guideline. If you are working skillfully, you should be able to stop in the middle of a conversation and have a sense of what you are doing, why, and how the patient is reacting to the structure you are providing and the strategy you have employed. This does not mean that the conversation should be full of flawless promises to change behavior. Indeed, you and the patient might be very confused about where to go next. But you should at least be aware that this is happening, and have a sense of where to go next in the consultation. You do not need to have all the answers about behavior change, but you should at least be able to manage the consultation. If confused, you can sometimes be frank with the patient to remarkably good effect.

Skillful practitioners are delinquent!

Practitioners might need to apply these strategies in a relatively mechanical way to begin with, much as one does when learning to drive. Things can feel clumsy and a bit forced. In these circumstances it would be unwise to blame yourself, or the strategies, if all that is happening is that you are learning about your and their potential and limitations.

We have noticed that, having taught these strategies to practitioners who practice them hard, they become delinquent! They get halfway through a strategy, leap onto another, return to where they left off, try something completely new, and so on. Observation soon reveals that this is creative adaptation of the highest caliber. Usually, however, they will say that they had some clumsy struggles to begin with. They will also report that the decision about what strategy to use next, often taken during a very brief pause in the conversation, requires more mental agility than the execution of the strategies themselves.

Skillful practitioners stick to simple things

Shortly before retiring, a hospital physician colleague said: 'Thirty years of experience has taught me to ask fewer questions, simpler questions and to listen very carefully to the answers'. This practitioner knew what simple open questions to use at the right time. Perhaps even more important, she apparently knew what to leave out, what was not essential to the fruitful conduct of the consultation. One colleague likened this process to the art of good cooking. His observation of a famous Chinese chef on television led him to observe, 'It all looks so easy, this cook just throws a few simple ingredients together. But it is deceptive. He knows what to leave out, and that must have taken a lot of practice' (Jeff Allison, personal communication).

Split yourself in half

It is obviously worthwhile to have your attention focused firmly on the patient. This is the art of active, empathic listening. You also need to have some of your attention focused on what is happening between the two of you, how the patient is reacting, and where you are at the level of strategy. This challenge is obviously not unique to talk about behavior change, but is an essential part of skillful helping and consulting of all kinds. You move along two trajectories at the same time.

CLINICAL ILLUSTRATIONS

Opportunistic health promotion: the example of smoking

Typical scenarios

You are a primary care practitioner. A patient has bronchitis and requests antibiotics. You know she is a heavy smoker.

You are a nurse conducting a chronic disease management clinic. A person with hypertension or diabetes attends for review: his condition is not well controlled and he continues to smoke.

Goals

- To make the most of the 'teachable moment' when established health problems are directly connected to unhealthy behaviors.
- To avoid alienating the patient by giving him or her yet another lecture.
- To avoid setting impossible goals so that the patient will inevitably harbor a sense of failure and frustration when he or she next visits.

- To maximize intrinsic motivation and to harness the patient's own ideas and resources for change.
- To realize that smoking is a major addiction that is influenced by a complex web of personal and social factors and which is unlikely to be overcome as a result of one brief consultation.
- Goals for the behavior change aspect of this consultation will vary according to the importance that individual patients place on change and their confidence in their ability to see it through. Simply planting a seed for change is a worthy achievement.
- To avoid being left frustrated by attempting to 'police' patients and failing to 'get people to change'.
- To provide the structure for individual patients to make effective decisions rather than trying to live their lives for them.
- Patient goals should be realistic and build on the patients' resources for change.

Principles and strategies

- Raise the subject in a non-threatening way which affirms a desire to understand the patient's position and respect for his or her decisions, even if these run counter to best medical wisdom.
- Explore how important giving up smoking is to the patient and enhance confidence in his or her ability to succeed in giving up.
- If importance is low, focus on that through asking useful scaling questions about importance score.
- Explore importance further by asking about pros and cons of smoking.
- Offer to share information in a non-judgmental way with those for whom giving up is not important. Keep the door open.
- If giving up is important to the patient but his or her confidence in succeeding is low, hone in on perceived barriers with useful scaling questions about increasing confidence.
- Taking the practitioner through a typical day in the patient's life will enhance rapport and invite the patient to make his or her own judgments about how he or she views his or her behavior.
- Brainstorm solutions to overcoming perceived barriers to successful quitting.
- Negotiate attainable goals.

Possible practice

Practitioner: *Yes, I agree you have bronchitis again. But it would help me get a better picture of your health if we could take a few minutes to talk about your smoking. I'm certainly not going to give you yet another lecture: today, my goal is to really try to understand a bit more about* *smoking from **your** viewpoint. OK? Won't you tell me what sort of smoker you are?*

The patient responds, usually briefly.

Practitioner: *I'm going to ask you two questions now that will help me understand things more clearly, and I want you to rate your answers on a scale. Firstly, how important is giving up smoking to you right now? If 1 is 'not at all important', and 10 is 'very important', what number would you give yourself right now?*

The patient thinks for a moment and gives a number.

Practitioner: *OK. Now I want to ask you about your confidence in your ability to quit and remain a non-smoker. If you did decide to try and quit, and 1 is 'not at all confident' and 10 is 'very confident' that you could give up and stay a non-smoker, what number would you give yourself now?*

If importance is low, ask any of the following useful questions:

You gave yourself a 3 for importance to you of giving up smoking. Why not 1?

Whatever basis there is for the person's motivation to change will now emerge. These have been called self-motivating statements (Miller & Rollnick 1991).

What would need to happen for you to move up from a 3 to a 6 or 7, say?

If confidence is the main problem, either of these kinds of question can be asked for confidence. An additional useful question is:

What can I, or we in this clinic, do to help you move up from a 3 to a 6 or 7?

If the practitioner feels that the patient is engaged and rapport is good, useful strategies could be tried.

When a sense of low importance is the main problem, the patient is usually feeling ambivalent; asking about the pros and cons of smoking may bring aspects of the patient's dilemma into sharp focus and the heightened tension from making the ambivalence so explicit may prompt serious consideration about change.

Building on the notion that it is better for patients to make their own evaluations, the practitioner invites the patient to say what he or she likes and dislikes about the behavior in question. After the patient has listed the positive sides, without interrupting or interpreting, the practitioner asks the patient to list the negative side of the coin as he or she sees it. The practitioner attempts to summarize both the pros and cons of the dilemma, keeping as closely as possible to the words used by the patient, and then asks the patient to say how the summary leaves him or her feeling and thinking. The practitioner should fight hard to avoid capitulating to inevitable urges to thump the tub of his or her own healthcare agenda.

Practitioner: *Tell me what you like about smoking?*

Patient: *You really want to know what I **like** about smoking? Gee, most people I've seen just give me the hell and damnation bit. Well now let's see, smoking definitely helps me relax, and in my job with all the uncertainty, I need that. I live a very stressful life you know. Funnily enough, smoking also gives me a feeling of giving something to myself, like it's my time for me. And I enjoy having a smoke when I have a drink with my friends.*

Practitioner: *OK, now tell me what you dislike about smoking?*

Patient: *Well, my wife nags me to hell and back, it does stink a bit, my kids hate it and sometimes I do worry about what it's doing to my lungs...*

Practitioner: *OK. So on the one had, you've got a stressful job and smoking gives you time for yourself, it helps you to relax and socialize. On the other hand, it stinks, and your family gives you a hard time about it, and sometimes you get worried about what it's doing to your health. Have I got it more or less about right? OK. Now, where does that leave you feeling right now about your smoking?*

Patient: *Well it certainly is a problem. I guess I've got to sit down and do some hard thinking.*

Another useful strategy is the Typical Day, where the practitioner asks the patient to think of a recent, typical day in his or her life and talk the practitioner through it, mentioning where the behavior in question fits in and how they felt about it. Again, the practitioner avoids the temptation to interrupt and extract lessons: the process of self-articulation is often a much more powerful teacher than external proselytizing. It also helps build rapport and engenders an understanding of the patient as a person. This interpersonal understanding and consequent sense of mutual respect can be a very powerful therapeutic tool.

For those patients for whom giving up smoking is not important right now, avoid nihilism. Research we conducted shows that the additional advantage of consulting in this style over brief advice is greatest among those whom practitioners assess as least ready to change (Butler et al, in press). And this is precisely the group that is least likely to receive opportunistic health promotion (Sesney et al 1997).

Offer to share information in a non-judgmental way. *Sure, it sounds like you are not ready to try to give up right now. That's fine. It's your decision and after all, no one else can make decisions for you. But I was just wondering whether some up-to-date medical information about the effects of smoking might help you in your decision making?*

Endeavor to couch information in general terms and then ask the patient to provide interpretations about his or her own specific circumstances. *The research into smoking shows that smoking does more damage among people with diabetes than those who do not have diabetes. On average, a 50-year-old smoker with diabetes will live an extra 3 years if he were to give up smoking. How do you interpret the implications of this for you?*

Most patients will say they already know all they want to know about the ill effects of smoking. As a rule, smokers are well informed about the negative health consequences of smoking, and a qualitative interview study we conducted shows that established smokers feel that that have already been saturated with a surfeit of anti-smoking information (Butler et al 1998).

The practitioner may say, *Fine, OK you know as much about the good and the bad sides of smoking as you feel you need to know. But can we agree to keep the door open on this one? Things often change and if you want to discuss the issue at any time, feel free to get in touch. By the way, did you hear about that 126-year-old woman in France who suddenly decided to give up smoking at the age of 112?*

For patients who feel that it is important to give up but who are low in confidence to succeed, *brainstorming solutions* can identify practical ways forward which are meaningful to the patient's unique situation.

Say a patient identifies fear of weight gain as his or her main barrier to giving up smoking. The practitioner may ask the patient to identify broad approaches to tackling this particular stumbling block. For example, one might ask, *What things do you know that people can do to lose weight?* Again, the practitioner encourages the patient to provide solutions and interpretations before offering suggestions of his or her own. Various general topic areas are identified, e.g. exercise, diet, drugs, eating less, eating differently, slimming clubs, and so on. The practitioner then asks, *Do any of these approaches appeal to you at the present time?* Again, the patient is encouraged to choose the approach that suits him or her best. He or she might say, *'Yes well, I could try eating differently.'* The practitioner again avoids jumping in with suggestions like, *Stop eating take-away meals or don't fry your food*, and instead asks the patient to identify the things he or she could do. Creative and surprising suggestions frequently emerge.

Giving lectures that set impossible goals for patients condemns both practitioners and patients to inevitable failure: *'Now I've told you before, and I am going to tell you again. By the time I next see you, you simply must have given up smoking, be eating only salads, have stopped drinking so much, and have started an exercise and relaxation program.'* Some chance! It is incumbent on the practitioner to ensure that the goals that patients select to work on are short-term and attainable: most patients with unhealthy behaviors have taken years to get into their present predicament, have been told many times to change, and have become accustomed to returning to the practitioner with an inbuilt sense of failure and sometimes resentment. Many see their visits to the doctor as a ritual in which they have to endure some admonishment before they can begin to express their own agenda. They are reminded of their failures, which harms their sense of self-efficacy and undermines their sense of themselves as a person who can make things happen, as opposed to being at the mercy of urges and stresses. But just as failure often begets failure, nothing breeds success like success; success more or less ensures that the patient will be able to come back next time with good news and this may be the first step in a new way of viewing themselves and the practitioner–patient relationship. Goals like agreeing not to increase the number of cigarettes smoked or taking the dog for a walk around the block twice a week can be the first small steps down a long road to healthier living.

Resistance will often rear its head: *Well doctor, I would love to give up smoking, I really would, but each time I try, I just about bite the kids' heads off. Even my husband says, 'For God's sake, go and have a cigarette if this is what giving up does to you'.* The thoughtless response is to say, *Well, I'm not going to collude with that. Of course giving up is tough. But after biting on the bullet for a week or two you'll get over it. Sometimes in life you've just got to stop making excuses and get down to business.* Such an approach is likely to damage the practitioner–patient relationship, and may even result in the patient changing doctors or not consulting when it would be appropriate to so. An alternative approach is agreeing with those aspects of the patient's comments that are accurate, and then to shift focus: *I know. For some people, giving up smoking can play havoc with their nerves. It really can be tough. I've seen people climb the walls, and I'm sorry that nicotine withdrawal affects you that way. But these days, there are treatments for that craving. They don't take it away, but they help take the edge off it. What do you know about nicotine replacement therapy, you know, the gum or the patches?*

This too may also be met with further resistance. *Well, I've tried the patches and they don't work for me.* or *It's too expensive.* or *I read a patient information leaflet about the patches, and all the side effects listed there made me terrified. I think I'm better off taking my chances smoking!*

Sometimes it seems that whatever the practitioner says will be countered by 'Yes but' in one form or another. This is a signal to avoid entering into a head-banging interaction where the smoker and practitioner 'Yes but' each other in a series of sterile encounters. Rather, move to closure, and use emphasizing personal choice or control as a good way of ending: *Sure. You get serious withdrawal symptoms and you have problems with nicotine replacement therapy. But giving up smoking remains the single most important thing you could do to improve your health now and to live a longer life. As you said earlier, that's important for you and your family. I agree one hundred percent that there are no easy ways to give up smoking. But at the end of the day, it's your life, and you have got to make some tough decisions for yourself. Nicotine replacement was just one suggestion. Maybe you could come up with a few of your own that might be better suited to your needs. After all, you are expert in what you want from life and what will or will not work for you when it comes to quitting smoking. I'll be around if you want to talk about ideas that you come up with at any time.*

Addressing multiple risk factors: the example of cardiac rehabilitation

Typical scenario

You are a cardiac rehabilitation specialist nurse. A patient attends after a diagnosis of stable angina was made. She drinks 35 units a week, is overweight, does very little exercise, smokes and just loves to eat fried foods.

Goals

- To maintain rapport with the patient. Change is likely to be a lifelong process and the patient will benefit from a trusting, supportive and understanding relationship with a practitioner.
- For the practitioner to accept that small shifts in attitude or taking a new look at an old problem is a worthy beginning.
- To promote an appropriate level of concern about risk (the patient should ideally be neither blasé nor so worried as to be incapacitated by anxiety).
- To avoid increasing resistance.
- To promote self-efficacy and responsibility.
- To view lifestyle holistically in that each aspect usually affects another: changing one unhealthy behavior may lead to change with another. However, keep the focus on practicalities rather than making global exhortations for dramatic sea changes in personality and behavior.

Principles and strategies

- Do not give the same patter to everyone. Target your information to the needs of the patient. Establish what the patient knows about the causes and course of his or her condition.
- Share information in language appropriate to the patient in a non-judgmental and non-threatening way.
- Sensitively raise the issue of lifestyle change.
- Use an agenda-setting chart to identify the patient's main current concerns and readiness to address each behavior.

- Assess importance and confidence for change when focusing on single behavior.
- Typical Day.
- Pros and cons.
- Brainstorming solutions.
- Negotiate attainable goals.

Possible practice

Practitioner: *I'm pleased you're feeling a bit better, and getting on OK with the tablets. But before we go on any further, I just want to say that the most important factor in your recovery will be how well you look after yourself. This depends on what you know about your condition. So I'd like to begin by checking what your information needs are, I want to check with you on your understanding of your condition.*

Patient: *Well, from what I gather, I've got a touch of angina. 'Stable angina.' Nothing too serious so long as I continue with the tablets.*

Practitioner: *What causes angina? What is happening inside your body?*

Patient: *It's a shortage of blood to the heart, or so they say. The heart is starved of oxygen a bit. Furring up of the arteries that takes the blood to the heart muscle, or something, by cholesterol. Nothing too serious.*

Notice the resistance emerging already (the patient is expressing skepticism), and notice too that the patient's level of anxiety about her condition, on the surface at any rate, is perhaps inappropriately low. Try a simple reflective listening statement: these are statements (not questions) which reflect the meaning of what the patient has just said. The practitioner's tone goes down at the end of the sentence. Such statements invite an explanatory response from the patient.

Practitioner: *Your angina, it's not too serious.*

Patient: *Well, lots of people have it, and I guess some do go on to have heart attacks. But mine is mild.*

Another reflective listening statement could be used at this point: *You might or might not have a heart attack yourself.* Or the practitioner could move to a direct question: *What do you understand of the causes of the problem? What could turn your mild angina into a very serious heart attack?*

Patient: *Well, they blame everything on smoking and they told me in the hospital that the smoking and the cholesterol brought this on and could make it worse. But heck, I don't smoke any more than most of my mates.*

Avoid this invitation to get into a resistance-enhancing argument by responding in a challenging way to this tantalizing but dangerous bait. 'Roll with the resistance.' Try agreement and a shift in focus to increase this patient's anxiety to an appropriate level.

> Practitioner: *You are 100% right! Angina is caused by the heart muscle being starved of oxygen by narrowed blood vessels, and smoking and cholesterol make it worse. Smoking is by far the most important thing that affects your condition right now. But it can also be made worse by being overweight, drinking too much, stress and not exercising. You are also right that your angina is mild at the moment. But there is nevertheless damage to your arteries, and it could get a lot more serious quite quickly. Changing some of the aspects of your life that lead to narrowing of the arteries could help you live a much longer, pain-free and active life.*

> Patient: *Yeah. But right now it's mild and under control.*

This patient continues to deny the seriousness of her problem. Amplified reflection is a strategy that could be tried here. The goal is to reflect back to the client in an amplified or exaggerated form. This should be done very carefully, avoiding sarcasm or hostility.

> Practitioner: *You should be able to get away without changing your lifestyle.*

> Patient: *No of course not! I really do want to stay healthy. I've got my job and family to think about.* (Notice that a self-motivating statement has at last emerged)

> Practitioner: (Emphasizing personal control) *Well, you're the boss here. It's your life. My job is to give you the information you need to help you make decisions which you feel are best for you and to provide support and help when you decide to change. I'm also concerned about you as one of my patients and as a human being with a condition which could become very serious quite quickly.*

> Patient: *Yeah, I know you're only trying to help, but I don't want anyone to nag me. The doctor who was in charge of my case when I was admitted in the hospital treated me like I was a naughty schoolgirl.*

> Practitioner: *No nagging, I promise. You're in the driving seat. I know it's useless me trying to make decisions for you and unfortunately neither of us is a schoolgirl any more! So I'm going to try something different now. Here is a chart* [practitioner produces agenda-setting chart] *which may help you in the process of thinking about aspects of your life that have a bad*

effect on your heart and which can improve your outlook if you change them. But notice here and here are some blank circles for you to put your own concerns into. Concerns that you may feel affect your health or which you just want to talk about. Which of these things, if any, do you feel ready to explore a bit further today?

Patient: *Well, I would like to do something about the way I eat.*

Practitioner: *OK, regarding the food issue, I'm going to ask you two specific questions which involve you rating yourself on a scale from 1 to 10. How important do you feel more healthy eating is to you right now? If 1 is 'not at all important', and 10 is 'very important', what number would you give yourself right now?*

Patient: *Nine or ten. Not only for my heart, but for my figure. Sometimes I feel I look like a slob. I deal with the public at work. I don't think looking like a slob helps me professionally.*

Practitioner: *How confident are you, again on a scale of 1 to 10, that you could make lasting changes to the way you eat? If 1 is 'not at all confident' and 10 is 'very confident', what would you give yourself right now?*

Patient: *Well zero while my partner does all the shopping and cooking. My partner is as thin as a beanpole regardless of what he eats, and he loves his food fried. Don't you just hate the type?*

Practitioner: *OK, so let's consider ways in which you could tackle this problem and get to eat more of what you would like to. What ideas have you got?*

Patient: *Well, I could kick him out. No, seriously, perhaps you could talk to him.*

Practitioner: *Sure, having a meeting with the three of us is one excellent way forward. Any other specific changes you could think of?*

Patient: *Well, I guess I could do the shopping and cooking if he could pick the kids up from school: that way I would be more in control of what we eat.*

Practitioner: *And how would you eat differently if you could get control of the shopping and cooking?*

Patient: *I could grill more, go for things like jacket potatoes every now and then, more fish. My friend is a vegetarian and she comes up with some good dishes without any meat at all.*

Practitioner: *Great. I can see you have some excellent ideas. So why don't we leave it there for now, and you can talk to your partner about the question of what you eat and how it could seriously affect what happens to your health. I'd be happy to meet with the two of you, if he feels that would help. I agree that serious change probably involves getting his help. And you will talk about him picking up the kids in exchange for you doing the shopping and cooking. How does that sound?*

The ongoing process of monitoring resistance and readiness is crucial in such consultations: the patient is coming to terms with the loss of aspects of his or her health, and adjustment is a complex and dynamic process. Different people will use varying strategies to deal with it, and the same person may change quite quickly in terms of how he or she reacts to bad news. In the foregoing scenario, the patient's defence was to minimize the problem. However, some patients will feel like they have received a death sentence and are frightened to embark on certain changes (e.g. exercising or having sex after a heart attack). Other patients will argue that there is no point in change since their condition is beyond palliation. So while the goal was to raise the level of anxiety in the above scenario, sharing information will be important to reduce anxiety in other patients who are too anxious to take practical steps for change.

Compliance

Many practitioners will recognize elements of the following scenarios in their clinical practice. While not specifically dealing with each scenario, what follows should generate some ideas which are relevant to all similar situations.

Typical scenarios

You are working in an outpatient clinic for people with epilepsy. A patient with frequent fits swears he is taking the medication as prescribed. Blood levels of the drug are consistently low. You increase the dose of his drug. The blood levels remain low. The patient says, 'I can't understand why my blood level is so low because I take my medicine as regular as clockwork, every night before I go to bed'.

You are a nurse in a clinic for people with diabetes. A patient with diabetes insists he is taking his medicine as prescribed and is sticking to his diet. When he attends for blood tests, the random sugar (a measure of short-term compliance) is always very low but the glycosylated hemoglobin (testing longer-term blood sugar levels) is very high. This suggests he takes his medicines only for those few days just prior to seeing you.

You are a nurse running a chronic disease management clinic for people with hypertension. A patient with hypertension attends faithfully, but despite numerous therapeutic changes and additions, his blood pressure has not changed. It did come down while he was in hospital receiving supervised treatment. The patient says, *'Blood pressure still up? Are you sure the doctor has prescribed the right tablets?'*.

You are a general medical practitioner in a busy surgery. The mother of a child with bad eczema wants a stronger steroid cream. She insists she is using oils in the bath and moisturizing creams all the time. Yet these were last prescribed over 8 months ago, and if used properly would have run out in a month.

Goals

- Not to alienate the patient or provoke resistance.
- To avoid being judgmental.
- To understand what medication means to patients in practical terms (hassle of using medication as prescribed) as well as in terms of their views of themselves (e.g. stigma).
- To be flexible and to negotiate. Patients have to make their own appraisals of risk and benefit and live with the consequences. Practitioners cannot take medicine for patients. The practitioner's job is to provide the structure and information for patients to make choices that are best for them.
- To make the treatment experience as user-friendly as possible.

Principles and strategies

- Raise the subject in an honest yet non-confrontational way: explain your confusion or puzzlement.
- Speak initially in general terms before putting the patient personally on the spot.
- Assess the importance to the patient of taking the medicines as prescribed.
- Promote the patient's confidence in his or her ability to take the medicine as prescribed.
- Use standard scaling questions.
- Check the patient's understanding of what is expected and how he or she is actually taking the medicine. The Typical Day strategy may be useful.
- If the problem is one of low personal importance, provide information in a non-judgmental way for the patient to factor into his or her decision making. The pros and cons strategy may be useful. If the problem is mainly confidence in implementing a decision to take the medicines, then brainstorm solutions.

• Negotiate attainable goals which are acceptable to both patient and practitioner.

Possible practice

Gary, I'm glad that you are feeling so well. I just want to be sure I know exactly when and what medicines you are using. Would you mind if we just spent a moment or two focusing on other aspects of the medication? Can I just ask you how important is taking the medicine to you right now? So that I can get a really accurate sense of what you feel: if 1 is 'not at all important', and 10 is 'very important', what number would you give yourself for how important taking the medicine is to you right now? ... Five! Excellent.

OK, say you did decide that taking your medicine was very important to you, how confident are you that you could begin and continue to take your medicine as prescribed? If 1 is 'not at all confident' and 10 is '100% confident' that you could stick to the regime exactly, what number would you give yourself right now? ... Five as well.

Let me ask you now, for importance of taking the medicine to you, you gave yourself a 5. Why not a 1?

I see, you feel medicine might help you in the long term, but what happens to you right now is more important. And right now the medicine makes you feel bad.

Right. You also gave yourself a 5 for confidence in your ability to take the medicine as prescribed. What would help you to move up from a 5 to say a 7 or 8?

Here, the patient may identify practical barriers in his or her daily life (e.g. inconvenience: taking inhalers while at work) and psychological barriers (e.g. stigma: a teenager with diabetes feeling an outsider when not able to drink a lot of alcohol with friends).

If little emerges to work on as a result of assessing importance and confidence, try a Typical Day: *Taking any sort of medication every day is tedious in anyone's language. There are very few people who like taking medicine, and yet it is an important part of controlling illness. And everyone is different in how taking medicine affects them and how they feel about it. It would help me to give the best input into your care if you would give me a clearer picture of how you feel about your medicine and how it fits into your life. A good way into this would be if you would think of a recent typical day in your life and take me through it, telling me when you use medicines and how you feel about it at the time. Take me through yesterday, for example.*

During this process, ask how the patient feels about him- or herself and the medicines. Fascinating insights commonly emerge. Taking medicines is often inconvenient and causes unpleasant side effects in ways the practitioner never imagined. It may also remind the patient of his or her loss of health, loss of control and of associated stigma. *Heavens above! With all that going on, it must be difficult to remember to take the medicine exactly as we doctors and nurses expect you to. You've certainly told me a thing or two that I hadn't thought about before, and I am at least beginning to understand what this illness means from your point of view. This can only help me in providing you with the best advice tailored to your unique circumstances so that you can make decisions about your own health which are right for you. After all, it's you that has to take (or not take) the medicines and it's you who has to live with the consequences.*

This could lead into asking about pros and cons. *OK, fine. You really miss that feeling that you are a normal, healthy human being, just like your mates, and that's especially bad when you go out with them on Saturday nights and when you go down to the beach for the weekend. Is there a way of taking some, if not all, of your medicine which might not interfere with your sense of who you are so much? Give me all your ideas, no matter how wild or crazy they may seem.*

Often the practitioner may find that the patient is already taking huge risks in any case and relatively simple advice and acceptance may diminish overall risk taking, even if exact compliance is not achieved. At least honesty is injected into the practitioner–patient relationship when suboptimal compliance can be discussed openly.

Patient: *You mean you wouldn't mind if I didn't test my sugars over the weekends, so long as I took a lower dose of my insulin on those days?*

Practitioner: *What I mind is not the issue here. What matters is how you feel and to get right the balance between your enjoyment of life, control of the illness now and possible long-term complications. All I am saying is that giving yourself a break over the weekends for the next while may mean that you look after yourself better during the week and overall. I'm prepared to support you if you want to give it a try, so long as we regularly reassess the situation. What do you think?*

Then negotiate acceptable, attainable goals: *So for the time being, you've decided to give yourself only one shot of long-acting insulin on Saturday mornings before you go out with your mates, and on these days you won't check your sugars. But on other days you'll stick with your twice-daily dosage as prescribed and also check your sugars. See me in a month and tell me how it goes.*

If low importance is the main problem, the pros and cons strategy is useful in bringing the decision dilemma into sharp, conscious focus. Often, compliance issues are pushed into the background of one's mind and although knowledge may be adequate, a kind of non-compliance by default occurs rather than through a considered, owned decision-making process. Pros and cons may also give the practitioner insights into the patient's information needs.

Arguing and denying are common features of consultations which focus on adherence to prescribed medication. As always, the practitioner should initially turn down the patient's invitation to an immediate boxing match in the consulting room. One way forward is simply explaining one's puzzlement to the patient. Where possible, frame contradictions in terms of generalities rather than in the individual's specific behavior. If possible, put the patient in the role of the problem solver, rather than the practitioner seeing him- or herself as a detective whose cunning has tripped the patient up. *Well, I don't understand it. You are taking your tablets and yet your blood levels are low. Most people on this dose of tablet will have a blood level of x. What do you think could be happening?* Or, *Gosh! It's 3 months since we last prescribed that inhaler for you. Most people use up those inhalers in half that time. What do you think could be happening to your asthma?* Or, *Most children get better using very little of the potentially dangerous steroid cream because they use a lot of the moisturizers on a regular basis. What do you think could be happening with your child?*

Low mood

Typical scenario

You are seeing a woman who has three school-going children. She tells you that she feels terrible and that she is not coping very well. Life seems just one big struggle. You know that improved mood often flows from the sufferer changing aspects of his or her everyday life, so recovery and behavior change are usually closely linked.

Goals

- To provide safe care, offering appropriate treatments which may involve other professionals. However, use your interaction to promote a sense of self-worth and control over at least some aspects of the world.
- To be supportive and empathetic, without colluding with defeatism.
- To negotiate goals which are more or less certain to be attained: assert the value of seemingly small achievements.
- To promote a shorter-term, day-by-day view of the process of recovery rather than setting daunting long-term goals.
- To ensure that expectations for recovery are realistic. The patient should expect slow progress as well as setbacks.

Principles and strategies

- Typical Day.
- Invite the patient to reflect on his or her daily achievements.
- Use a modified agenda-setting chart.
- Assess importance and confidence for embarking on an alternative, control-enhancing strategy.
- Brainstorm solutions.
- Negotiate short-term, attainable goals.

Possible practice

Where new, therapeutic behaviors have not yet been identified by either party in the consultation, to begin with assessing importance and confidence to change is not appropriate. Typical Day is a better place to start, since it provides a direct route into the patient's physical symptoms, her psychological state and the contextual modifying factors. This bio-psychosocial approach to diagnosis and treatment is especially important in patients with a mood disorder.

> Practitioner: *I wonder if I could ask you to tell me a little more about your life and the problems you are coping with right now? It would help me to understand the situation better if you could pick a typical day in your life, say like yesterday, and take me through it from when you woke up. Tell me about the things you struggled with and how you felt at the time.*

The patient may need further encouragement and brief prompting to give the practitioner a picture of her day, the problems that arose and her feelings at each hurdle. As the story unfolds, it is likely that the practitioner will gain an in-depth knowledge of the patient's level of function, variation in mood states throughout the day, view of the future, existing coping strategies, support base, and contributing external factors to the low mood. Assessments of danger to self in this way (possibility of deliberate self-harm) may be more sensitive than traditional direct questioning, since an account of a typical day will provide a more accurate assessment of the frequency and intrusiveness of such thoughts. The practitioner is often left with a genuine sense of the enormous effort that a patient in such a position is making to get through each day. Several important achievements in this day's struggle are likely to emerge which the patient could rightly feel proud of. The practitioner may simply ask the patient to identify and then reflect on such apparently small achievements.

> Practitioner: *Great. Now I really can see what you mean when you say that life is a huge struggle for you at the moment. I can see that there are some things that you have handled in a way which frustrates you. But I must*

say, given how you are feeling, there are things you told me that I, for one, was deeply impressed by. Perhaps you could list the things that you realize you handled well?

That's excellent! When one is feeling low, it's common not to be able to identify anything positive about oneself, and forcing yourself to list not only the negative but also the positive things, no matter how apparently trivial they might seem, is an important discipline to nurture as one begins a journey down the road to feeling better. At the end of each day, listing such achievements, no matter how small, may help to get the day in better perspective. I have to say that given how bad you are feeling, I am deeply moved by how hard you are trying to keep things going and how much you are succeeding in achieving. I know you are very irritable; your shouting at the kids worries you and sometimes you feel you just can't go on. But somehow you do carry on. As you say, the facts that you get three kids off to school each day and are there for them when they come back, you feed them, you give them care, attention and love and you get them to bed are significant aspects of your day, any of which anyone could justifiably feel proud of. One just has to go through a day like that once to know how exhausting it can be.

Now let's tackle the more frustrating things that you mentioned. I am going to draw a few circles on this blank page and I'll write each frustration that you mentioned in a circle. We call this thing an agenda-setting chart. OK, so here we've got poor sleep, here screaming at the kids, here housework, not doing anything to relax and finally smoking too much. I want you to select one of these to work on in the next while. Try to choose something that you feel reasonably able to tackle right now ... Whew! That's brave! Screaming at the kids in the morning! That is a serious problem at a time when I know you are feeling at your worst and at your most helpless.

Assess importance and confidence in change. Importance is likely to be high and confidence low.

Practitioner: *You mentioned that not shouting at the kids in the mornings is very important to you but you are not confident you can manage to change. OK, so what ideas have you got for improving this aspect of your day? ... Great. As you say, you could get up a bit earlier and prepare things a bit more before they come down and, as you say, you could explain to them the night before that things are difficult for you. Some day you might give them each a specific task to help get the day going smoothly. That will take a while, I agree, to get them into the routine and to know you mean business, but if you could pull it off somewhere down the line, that would be a major achievement. But for the moment, why don't we begin with you waking up 15 minutes earlier and getting things ready before they come down? That way, when they are there, you might feel more relaxed and in control.*

Say the patient chose to build some quality relaxation time into her day. The practitioner might not even assess importance and confidence since he or she may already have a good feel for these two domains.

Practitioner: *So, the time in the middle of the day that right now you spend on your own when you feel worst, when thoughts of all the problems come flooding into your mind. Is there anything active you can think of that you might enjoy doing during this time? ... Going for a walk if the weather is fine, seeing a friend, taking in a movie, spoiling yourself at the shops: sure, all good suggestions ... Is there a goal that you would like to set for yourself in this regard? ... Great! Why don't we say that for at least one day this week you might go out for a walk in the middle of the day?*

Summarizing is important both to ensure a common understanding of the goals, but also to ensure that there is agreement about what is expected.

Practitioner: *Excellent. So to summarize, at the end of each day, as I understand it, you have agreed to make a deliberate effort to routinely consider the things you did OK and well, and not to think about just the things that disappoint you. It might even be a good idea to write your positive achievements down in list form at the end of each day. Secondly, you are going to try to get up a little earlier to prepare for the kids so that you can feel more in control when they come down (or one day in the week, you might go out for a walk on your own). Is that how you see what we agreed? Do you feel these goals are manageable?*

Patient: [Putting her head in her hands] *All this is easy for you to say. I'm the one who has to do it.*

This resistance may take the practitioner slightly by surprise and would not have become apparent had the practitioner not checked back with the patient. The unthinking response is to say, *Listen, all I'm trying to do is to help you make a program to enable you to help yourself. You have to get moving on this one!* This may make the patient feel badgered and even more defeated. When response to goals is less than enthusiastic, it could be that importance and confidence have been misassessed and it is worth checking back. In this case, confidence is clearly the main issue.

Practitioner: *I know that life is tough for you right now. Perhaps I have underestimated exactly how difficult it is for you to make changes right now. How confident are you that you could make a list each day of your achievements and get up 15 minutes earlier to get ready for the kids?*

Patient: *I don't know. It takes me so long to get to sleep. I do my best sleeping at the end, you know, just before I wake. The thought of getting up earlier just makes me feel sick, even though I know it might help with the kids.*

Practitioner: *That's fine. Keeping the list: how confident are you that you could do that?*

Patient: *The list I think I could manage.*

Practitioner: *Good. The important thing is that you make a start, and I feel that keeping a list of all your achievements each day is an excellent beginning. Will you show it to me when we meet again?*

End with a supportive statement and a note of realistic optimism.

Practitioner: *Now just before we part, I want to say that it has taken a while to get to feeling so bad. Getting to where you would like to be will not be easy and you will have many setbacks along the way. But by focusing on small things and looking at the next step rather than the whole journey, I'm confident that things will gradually improve. Doubtless, there will be some days on which you feel back at square one, but as time goes by, these episodes generally last a shorter and shorter time for people who are beginning to take control of their low mood. So let's meet up in a fortnight and you can let me know how you got on with the goal you set today.*

The content of the goals is less important than ensuring that there is some sense of achievement built into the next meeting. The crucial switch is for this patient to develop a sense of herself as someone who can to some extent at least control her situation, rather than seeing herself as simply reacting to events.

Promoting safer sexual practices

Typical scenarios

You are a nurse working in a family planning clinic. Your next patient says, 'I've got a regular partner now and I'd like to be on the pill'.

You are a doctor in a genitourinary medicine clinic. A patient asks you about a rash on his penis. He tells you he is gay.

Goals

- To develop a trusting relationship where frank discussion about sensitive issues is comfortable.
- To maintain reasonable boundaries and avoid excessive intimacy.
- To enhance knowledge of safe sex and promote low-risk sexual behavior.
- To enhance the patient's sense of being in control and of being able to say 'no' in an uncomfortable situation.

Principles and strategies

- Raise health promotion issues sensitively.
- Establish the patient's information needs.
- Avoid giving a lecture.
- Assess importance and enhance confidence to practice safe sex.
- Use scaling questions.
- Try eliciting the pros and cons of an aspect of the practice of safe sex.

Possible practice

Practitioner: *Sure, I'm happy to prescribe the pill and act as a resource for you on contraception and sexual health more generally. I appreciate the fact that you have taken this responsible step to come and talk about it all. We'll go through the more medical aspects of the pill in a minute, but would you mind if we first discussed some of the wider implications of being sexually active first? ... To save me gabbling on about things you already know, can I ask you to tell me a bit about what being sexually active means to you as a person?*

Patient: *I feel I'm ready for it now, and it's something I want to be able to do. But I do get a bit worried. Well, Mark wanted me to go on the pill ... he doesn't always like using condoms and sometimes we just don't. I get worried ... and they are such a hassle.*

Practitioner: *Could we spend a moment talking a bit about condoms? Using condoms is crucial to the practice of safe sex, especially if you are not in a long-established relationship. How important is using condoms to you right now? I'm going to be quite specific and ask you to rate its importance to you on a scale of 1 to 10. If 1 is 'not at all important' to you and 10 is 'very important', what number would you give yourself right now?*

Patient: *Well, I don't want to catch anything bad. I'm young and want to stay healthy, so I'd give myself a 9.*

Practitioner: *OK. Now how confident are you that you could practice safe sex every time you make love? Again, if 1 is 'not at all confident' and 10 is 'very confident', what number would you give yourself right now?*

Patient: *Gee, perhaps a 5 or 6. Mark doesn't like to use them, and I'm not wild about them either. Mark sometimes seems to think I don't trust him if I ask him to put on a condom. Nothing bad has happened yet.*

Practitioner: *So you would like to use condoms all the time but it's not always easy to do. What would help you to move from a 5 to a 10, and practice safe sex every time you made love?*

Patient: *It's Mark, I guess. I find it difficult to insist sometimes. I'd need him to be more supportive.*

Equally, the practitioner could leave out the numbers and ask the importance and confidence questions in his or her own style. *How important do you feel using condoms is for you in your life right now?* or *How confident are you in your present situation that you could make sure you always had condom-protected sex?*

Returning to the problem of asserting her views with her partner, the practitioner may say: *Do you think you could talk to him about it at a time when you are not about to make love?*

Patient: *Well, it is difficult. But if there is something on the television about sex, perhaps we could talk then.*

Practitioner: *Do you want to run through with me the kinds of things you would say as a kind of rehearsal? So when you do raise it you've got all you want to say in your mind.*

Patient: *Well I want to tell him that I want to use condoms not because I don't trust him, but because its something that everyone should be doing. I heard a talk about it. Stamping out AIDS and keeping my chances open for having a baby later.*

Practitioner: *Great! As you say, it's something all people in your situation should be doing. Now let's get onto the pill itself. What do you think about using both a condom and the pill early on in relationships?*

This patient had a high importance score and a lower confidence score. Using pros and cons might have worked with someone to whom practicing safe sex was less important. For example:

Practitioner: *You gave yourself only a 2 or 3 for importance to you of using condoms. Perhaps you could tell me what you dislike about using condoms and then say what you think is good about using condoms every time you have sex?*

Patient: *I don't like using them because I feel sex is less natural, the sensation is, you know, less, and asking your partner to put on a condom can spoil the moment: like taking a cold shower!*

Practitioner: *OK, tell me what might be good about using condoms?*

Patient: *Well, I know that it might cut down my chances of getting AIDS and other infections. But that's it.*

Practitioner: *So on the one hand it's more natural without a condom, and putting one on can spoil the magic of sex and it's not always easy to ask your partner to put one on. On the other hand, using a condom could save you from getting infected with the HIV virus and getting other diseases like gonorrhea. So where does that leave you in your thinking about using condoms now?*

Resistance may take many forms. Most people underestimate their risk of being infected compared to their understanding of the risks to others.

The practitioner may ask: *Can I just check back with you on one thing. What do you know about the risks of unsafe sex? What are your chances of getting infected with HIV?*

Patient: *Well, with better treatments available these days, HIV may soon be a curable infection.*

The practitioner may try simple reflection. This is best done in the form of a simple statement: *You're not worried about getting HIV.*

Patient: *I'm not saying that. Of course I'm worried about getting HIV. Only a fool would not be worried about getting HIV …* (Self-motivating statements begin to flow)

Patient pressures on practitioners to prescribe medicines which are not indicated on biological grounds

This is an example where practitioners would prefer not to meet patients' stated needs largely for clinical reasons.

Typical acute prescribing scenario

You are a primary care physician. Your patient has a sore throat that is almost certainly caused by a virus. 'Yes doctor, you have told me all that before. I know it's probably a virus. Can I have my antibiotic now please.'

Typical long-term prescribing scenarios

You work in a pain clinic. You are trying to suggest pain management strategies which do not involve strong compound analgesics. 'That is all very well for you to say doctor, but you don't have to live with the pain. I need my prescription.'

You are working in a psychiatry outpatient department, and see someone who has been on tranquilizers for many years. You raise the subject of the tranquilizers. 'Of course I would prefer not to take the tranquilizers. I'm not really a 'pill person'. But I do need them every now and then. Can I have a full month's supply this time? It'll save me having to bother you so often.'

Goals

- To practice ethically by avoiding prescribing medicines which are of dubious biomedical benefit.
- To encourage patient empowerment by promoting a sense of responsibility for negotiated decisions.
- To at least sow a seed that there are also non-pharmacological ways of coping with the discomfort the patient is experiencing.
- To preserve the doctor–patient relationship.
- To minimize the practitioner's sense of frustration.
- To ensure that the patient feels listened to, supported and understood.

Principles and strategies

- Assess importance to the patient of a low drug approach and enhance confidence to change.
- Consider how far it is possible and desirable for the practitioner to meet the patient's request on this occasion.
- Hand over as much control as possible to the patient.
- Elicit reasons which are real for the patient about the merits and otherwise of taking the medicines.
- If importance is low, engage in non-judgmental information sharing.
- Use pros and cons strategy with ambivalent patients.
- When importance is high and confidence is low, use brainstorming solutions to identify solutions.
- Set attainable goals.

Possible practice: acute medication

How many times are explanations about the inappropriateness of drugs in specific situations met with a dogged determination to get the drug from the doctor, sometimes at all costs? Under these conditions, it is tempting for the practitioner to grit his or her teeth and either issue the prescription or become challenging. The former solution usually leaves the practitioner feeling frustrated and nothing really changes for the patient. The second response increases the practitioner's blood pressure and provokes resistance in the patient.

Let us explore more creative ways out of this situation with the help of the example of a mother who wants antibiotics for what is almost certainly a viral infection in her child. First, try to establish the importance of a non-antibiotic approach to the mother.

> Practitioner: *I'm not saying I'm not going to prescribe antibiotics under any circumstances, but I feel this is an important decision and we should take it very seriously. Everyone has their own views on the topic, and I want to be sure that I properly understand yours. So that I can be sure that I know how you feel about antibiotics in situations like this, I want to begin by asking you how important antibiotics are for you in this situation.*

> Patient: *Well, I know they work for me when I get like this, and we've never had problems from them before. I need the antibiotics. That is why I have come all this way to see you.*

Assessing confidence in implementing a non-antibiotic approach is probably not worthwhile in the face of such importance the patient attaches to taking antibiotics now. Generally, if the importance of change is very low, always address that before exploring confidence.

Here we have a situation where the patient and practitioner are on opposite ends of the importance spectrum. When it comes to taking antibiotics for this condition, this patient rates importance highly and this practitioner rates it as low. Changing this person's perception of the importance of antibiotics in this situation while preserving the practitioner–patient relationship in a single consultation may not be possible. A more realistic goal is to be sure that the patient understands that the best medical wisdom is clear that taking antibiotics will not help her get better quicker and that the antibiotics carry dangers for which the patient will have to share responsibility. Perhaps then a seed will be sown and next time, and perhaps next year, the patient will be prepared to at least consider ways of dealing with these infections which do not involve antibiotics.

One way of approaching this situation is to say, *I understand your concerns and I will give you the antibiotics this time if that is what you feel is best. However, I would not be doing my job as a doctor if I did not first share with you some concerns. There is a lot of research on many thousands of patients which shows that people with coughs and clear lungs do not benefit from taking antibiotics. The drugs carry a risk of side effects. What do you make of this research?*

If the patient is not ready to engage, the practitioner may wish to honestly state his or her position and move to closure, emphasizing personal choice and responsibility. *Well, research shows that antibiotics will probably do no good in situations like this. They could even do some harm which can occasionally be life-threatening. Do you know of any dangers associated with antibiotics? … Well there are some dangers which you should know about. Minor side effects like upset stomachs and rashes are common, and serious reactions like bone marrow problems and allergies do sometimes occur. Using antibiotics also makes bugs resistant to them, which could mean that when you really need them for a life-threatening infection, they don't work so well. Today, this decision is ultimately yours. First consider all the downsides and the fact that antibiotics in this situation are unlikely to do you any good. Then if you feel that on balance, taking them is right for you now, go ahead.*

Some patients will be aware that antibiotics are a mixed blessing, and might be more ambivalent. Here, one may try a pros and cons strategy: *You feel that you probably need antibiotics in this situation. Fair enough, you are the expert when it comes to how you feel now and how you have been helped by these drugs in the past. I wonder though, have you heard about some of the problems that can be caused by antibiotics? So that we can be sure that I understand your thinking in this regard, perhaps you could quickly tell me some of the reasons why you think antibiotics are appropriate now and some of the reasons why they might not be?*

Some patients will feel that it is very important to try alternatives to drug treatment, but are worried how they will manage (low in confidence). Exploring the importance of doing without antibiotics is obviously less critical among these people. Practitioners are likely to get more returns for their efforts if they focus on building confidence to cope differently. Suggesting practical strategies will be useful. In the case of the request for antibiotics for sore throats, one might elicit ideas from the patient and then suggest the use of fluids, antipyretics and analgesics if these have not yet been mentioned. Offer to review the patient within a day, or give the patient a prescription for an antibiotic but ask him or her not to take the drug unless symptoms deteriorate.

Possible practice: long-term medication

In the case of chronic analgesic or benzodiazepine use, one can offer a very slow program of change where the patient is in the driving seat and the practitioner provides ongoing support. The underlying problem is often a chasm between how the two parties in the consultation view solutions. The patient often wants a biomedical, simple solution while the practitioner sees the situation as a chronic problem best addressed through lifestyle adjustment.

Practitioner: *Sure, I'll definitely give you your medication, but I just want to ask you a bit more how you feel about using this amount of dihydrocodeine? Right now, how important to you is cutting down on the amount of painkillers you are using? If 1 is 'not at all important' and 10 is 'very important', what number would you give yourself right now?*

OK, and how confident are you that you could cut down if that was your decision? If 1 is 'not at all confident' and 10 is 'very confident' that you could cut down and keep on with less medicine, what number would you give yourself right now?

You gave yourself 8 for importance to you of cutting down. Why not 1?

Patient: *Well Doc, I don't like taking medicines. I know they are addictive and I would like to be well again, off all the pills.*

Practitioner: *What would help your confidence in your ability to cut down and move up from a 4 to an 8 or 9?*

If the patient was able to come up with suggestions, the process of brainstorming solutions might continue from here. If the patient was not able to come up with many practical suggestions, try using Typical Day and then move into brainstorming solutions.

Practitioner: *Changing established patterns of medicine use is never easy, and I applaud your courage in agreeing to experiment with whether you can do with less. I want you to be the main decision maker here. We will move at your speed, and I will encourage you to go slowly and to expect setbacks. I will be here to support you in the decisions you make. Now let's see, at the moment you are using 10 tablets of dihydrocodeine a day. Take me through a typical day in your life, telling me when your pain gets bad and when you use the tablets. I also want you to think about what else you could have done apart from taking the tablets.*

Good. I think this has been very useful for me. You have helped me understand the intensity of the pain and the courage you are already showing in managing it. (Practitioners who have heard the detail of the daily lives of their patients will seldom fail to be moved by their accounts of chronic pain or anxiety states and can usually make comments like this with absolute sincerity.) *What other options do you have say when the pain gets bad after lunch?* (Practitioner listens carefully to patient's suggestions and then may add one or two of his own.) *Right, so you could take a tablet, you could do something about the house to get your mind off it, you could take the dog for a walk around the block or you could have a hot bath. Which one of these options do you think you could go for over the next month? Great, so you reckon you could try and go for a short walk after lunch when the pain gets bad instead of taking a pill. How about we set a goal of, say, using 10 pills less (say 290 rather than 300) over the course of the next month and when we meet again, you can tell me how it's been going, walking the dog instead of using a pill on some days after lunch?*

Resistance can manifest in almost every conceivable form in these often fraught situations, for example **anger**: *I'm fed up with being told I don't need these tablets. I do, I tell you. I'm the one who has to live with this constant hell every day of my life,* **splitting**: *Doctor X told me I should never be without these tablets,* **challenging**: *You say these tablets can do harm. They are the only thing that has ever helped me,* **disagreeing**: *I would love to be able to cut down on my tablets. But there is nothing else that works,* and so on.

Key to dealing with resistance is convincing the patient that you share the same goals, namely to improve the patient's health. You are acting out of concern and commitment to the patient, not vindictiveness. Establishing this can be the springboard to shifting the focus off biomedical cures to considering personal and social components which affect the patient's suffering. Agreement about the seriousness of the patient's symptoms and then shifting focus is one way of concluding such consultations and opening the door to non-pharmacological approaches at the next visit.

Practitioner: Slow down! No one is talking of abandoning you without any medication or indeed in making changes that you are not ready for. All I'm doing is sharing with you research findings that long-term medication like this can cause some harm. Remember, I'm your doctor and I have a duty to inform all patients about the risks of medicines that I prescribe. I'm focusing on this issue not because I want to be nasty. Quite the opposite. I believe we have exactly the same goals here. We are both interested in you living a happier, healthier life. I see my role as helping you to make decisions which are right for you rather than telling you what to do. Now I believe you one hundred percent when you tell me how terrible you feel without your tranquilizers. Anyone who experiences those kind of feelings would want tablets that relieved their symptoms. But it also seems that you feel pretty bad sometimes even when you take the medication. Now I'm committed to working with you on this one. I just feel you can feel better, with or without tablets if you also focus on other things that are relevant to how you feel. Let's set aside the question of cutting down the tablets for the moment then, and talk about some of the things that influence your anxiety, other than tablets.

Patient: *Come off it. I know you just want to take my tablets away from me.*

Again, just be honest and try reframing the problem.

Practitioner: *Look, I make no secret of the fact that I am concerned about the medication. But that's not the only thing I am concerned about. I am concerned about how you feel. Tablets are only a small part of your life. Looking at tablets in relation to you as a whole person in order to help you feel better overall is my goal.*

Seeking unlikely cures: patients with no identifiable physical cause for their chronic discomfort and who want further tests

Typical scenario

You are a primary care practitioner. You look at the fat file in front of you and sigh. Fifteen years of pain, numerous rounds of expensive and some-times dangerous investigations. A human being mutilated by surgeons who have cut this and then that organ out of her in a desperate attempt to 'do something'. But still the pain goes on. Yip, Mrs Smith again. You know exactly what she will say to you even before you have called her into the consulting room: it has happened so many times before. 'Doctor, I know all the tests are negative and in the hospital they said I should see a psychia-trist. But I'm telling you, this kind of pain is not in my head. Surely that new scan I've heard about will be able to identify what's gnawing inside me? If only you would help me sort this pain out, I could start living my life again.'

Goals

- To promote acceptance in both the patient and the practitioner that the patient has taken years to get where she is: improvement is likely to occur only slowly.
- Investing a bit of extra time and emotional energy during this visit may cause a shift in attitude to the problem on the part of either or both parties.
- For the practitioner to accept that medicine 'cures' very few problems. A worthy goal is to help people accept and make the most of their imperfect situations and to initiate an approach which does not seek only biomedical solutions to discomfort and distress.
- Never to leave the patient feeling abandoned. Preserve hope, but keep this realistic and do not mislead the patient. Offer to see the patient regularly at structured intervals.
- To aim towards an acceptance that there is no magic bullet that will cure the patient. A quick fix is not on the cards. The next best thing is

adjusting goals from finding a cure to maximizing control over the symptoms.

Principles and strategies

- Try to see this old problem with fresh eyes: we often think we understand our patients and therefore we spend less time exploring beyond the biomedical to include personal and contextual considerations.
- Typical Day is often a good place to start in situations where new, alternative behaviors are not yet clearly articulated in the minds of either the patient or the practitioner.
- Information exchange.
- Pros and cons of having further tests at this time.
- Importance and confidence of alternatives to further medical tests.
- Watch resistance closely: assess personal control and consider agreement with a shift in focus.
- Keep an open mind; be flexible and negotiate.
- Set attainable goals.

Possible practice

Practitioner: *Good morning, Mrs Smith. Good to see you again. How are things going?*

Patient: *Not very well at all. I really am trying hard not to bother you and sometimes I feel you must be getting fed up with me and my ongoing problems. But I really think it's getting worse and I can't go on like this. My life is consumed by this pain, and all I want is to be well again. Now I was reading in a magazine about a man who had pain just like me and the doctors had also told him it was all in his head. Then he had a new, enhanced NMR scan and they found out what it was. They caught it just in time. Now I know I've had the NMR scan, but it wasn't the new, enhanced scan. What do you think about me having the new, enhanced scan?*

Saying 'no' to the new, enhanced scan at this stage would be akin to putting on a pair of boxing gloves. Try agreeing and then shifting the focus.

Practitioner: *OK, sure, the enhanced scan is definitely worth thinking about. Anything that could possibly help you live a fuller life deserves careful consideration. I see myself 100% as your advocate when it comes to tests and treatments. By that I mean it's my role to help you decide what is likely to help you and indeed what could harm your recovery. There are very few tests that do not have side effects. So before we make any decision about further tests, I want to be sure I have a complete picture in my mind so I can give you the best possible advice. I want to know about the exact nature of your symptoms and how they affect your life. Often, going over it all again in some detail can shed important light on the subject that I may have forgotten about. Who knows, you might give me new clues about the cause of the problems that I hadn't picked up before. It would help me a lot if you would think of a typical day in your life (say yesterday or the day before) and take me through it, beginning when you woke up, and telling me how you feel as you move through the day.*

Patient: *Well, I've kind of been through this before, and I can tell you right now you are not going to get me to see a psychiatrist.*

The client has created a massive block to engaging with the practitioner and participating in the Typical Day strategy. Agreement and expressing support for the patient in the face of major stumbling blocks can have profound results.

Practitioner: *Fine. No problem. Let's agree on that right now then. No psychiatrists! It's very important for me that you understand that I believe this pain is very serious and real to you. I have absolutely no doubt that your suffering is severe and real. The last thing I want to do is to send you off to yet another doctor. I am committed to the two of us doing our best to getting to grips with this problem together, and I want to assure you that I will stand by you in this process. But I do need your help. Telling me about a typical day in your life will help us make the best plans about your treatment together.*

Patient: *OK, I guess. Well, as I've said, I wake up with the pain in my abdomen; as I've said, there is also a full feeling and a pressing feeling on my spine, and then the pain builds up and up while I'm dressing, so I take my tablets which don't really help and then I go to the toilet which does ease it a bit but I'm never free of it. Then I try and eat something, otherwise my husband nags me. That usually makes it worse but I do it to keep him quiet. Then he goes off to work and leaves me with the pain…*

Practitioner: *How do you feel at this time?*

Patient: *Sometimes when he goes off I just want to put my head in a pillow and scream … to be honest, sometimes I do. Sometimes I feel that no one understands what I'm going through. How can they?*

The practitioner should avoid invitations to be sidetracked into anything else than the patient's account of her journey through a typical day.

Practitioner: *What happens next?*

The practitioner listens and asks further questions about how the patient feels at key points. Eventually, the practitioner may ask the patient to reflect on the relationship between her pain, its immediate context and her feeling at the time. *Mrs Smith, what you've told me will be invaluable to the process of decision making that we are both working on. I'm just wondering, are you able to identify patterns in your pain, for example times when your pain is worse or better, and what is going on in your life at the time?*

If the patient is not forthcoming, the practitioner may throw in an invitation to reflect on the loneliness she feels in her suffering. *Are there any things you could change which might make you feel more understood and less isolated in your pain?* Remember, in situations like this, radical change is not likely after one interaction along these lines. This patient's journey towards a view of the problem that is not focused purely on biomedical solutions and which incorporates acceptance of pain and adapting to life with pain is likely to be long and hard. Planting a seed for looking at the problem as one of adaptation rather than cure is perhaps the most realistic goal of this consultation.

Practitioner: *OK, excellent, well that is a start and I am sure that you might come up with further ideas later. But now I want to turn back to the question of the new, enhanced scan. … Why don't we quickly make a list of all the tests you've had, all the specialists you've consulted and all the operations you've undergone? … Good. What does all that say to you? … Yip. I agree. Its been a terrible journey of hope followed by disappointment, like searching for the holy grail or something, and you are right, modern medicine has not done a lot for you. But I just want to say that medicine is an imperfect thing. With all the things we see on television, it does sometimes leave both doctors and patients with a feeling that medicine should have all the answers. But the harsh reality is that it doesn't. I agree, no one has been able to cure you. And I think you're also saying that every time things got a little bit worse, your family doctor referred you for another scan which never really got to the bottom of things? And every time you saw another specialist, he did another test or cut another piece out of your body and still your symptoms did not change much? … I really am amazed at how much modern medicine has put you through for so little improvement in your pain.*

The practitioner could capitalize on the rapport established through this genuine exposition of concern and try a modified pros and cons strategy.

Practitioner: *Turning again to the new, enhanced scan, I want you to try and think of some of the advantages of having the scan, and then I want you to try and tell me about some of the reasons why a scan might not be the best option right now.*

Patient: *Well, doctor, the most obvious thing is that the scan might find out what is causing my pain, and once we know, we may be able to cure it. On the other hand, it could be like all the others: a lot of trouble and radiation for little benefit to me. To tell you the honest truth, I'm sick of going back and forwards to the hospital. I think they see me coming and say, 'Oh no, here she comes again', but I tell you, it's their fault. If they had taken me seriously in the first place I wouldn't be like this now.*

The patient is diverging from the pros and cons strategy and beginning to engage in a blaming exercise. This diverts energy away from the patient as the most important factor in shaping the future. Pinpointing fault is impossible and usually fruitless. The practitioner therefore avoids any discussion about blame.

The practitioner might provide some generalized information and ask the patient to interpret: *I was reading in a medical journal the other day about people who have had numerous operations over the years without any improvement in their symptoms. They found that discovering a physical cause for the pain that could be put right almost never happened with such people. The people who did best were those who started finding their own solutions rather than continuing to look to medicine to cure them. What do you make of this research?*

If this leads nowhere, endeavor to reinforce the implicit message, while at the same time expressing concern and flexibility. Remember, if this patient leaves your office dissatisfied, she will find another doctor who will send her for the scan and when her symptoms are not relieved, this new doctor is likely to tire of her and she will move on, trapped in a perpetual cycle of hope and disappointment and never seeing beyond the false grail of a biomedical quick fix.

Practitioner: *OK, well, like you, I can see good and bad sides to the scan. Now I'm not saying that I won't refer you for the scan under any circumstances, and I want you to know that I will do my best to provide you with the finest ongoing medical care. But I want to see the thing in perspective and see you as a whole person, not just as a collection of symptoms. Sometimes taking time out from the ongoing saga of tests and trying to answer the question, 'How can I live with the problem a little better?' as opposed to finding an absolute cure can be a good thing. But let's both keep an open mind. Returning to your pain, I wonder if we could make a list of some of the things that are associated with it being a bit worse and some of the things that you can do which seem to ease it a bit?*

Here the practitioner may use a modified agenda-setting chart, where things which are to a certain extent at least under the patient's control (e.g. tablets, communication with her partner, exercise, diet, distractions) are put in blank circles. Simply listing things that the patient could be in control of may be therapeutic in itself. The patient then selects one area to work on. Importance and confidence are then assessed in relation to this behavior, which could lead into using the useful scaling questions, brainstorming solutions and setting attainable goals.

Practitioner: *Why don't we leave it at that then for today. What you have told me today confirms in my mind how hard you are trying to cope with a bad situation. I like your idea of talking to your husband about your pain each day for about 5 or 10 minutes only, and then making sure that you have quality time together to talk and plan about other things which have nothing to do with your pain. Let me know how this has gone when we meet again in a fortnight.*

REFERENCES

Butler C C, Pill R, Stott N C H 1998 A qualitative study of patients' perceptions of doctors' advice to quit smoking: implications for opportunistic health promotion. British Medical Journal 316:1878–1881

Butler C C, Rollnick S, Cohen D, Russell I, Bachmann M, Stott N (in press) Motivational consulting versus brief advice for smokers in general practice: a randomised trial. British Journal of General Practice

Miller W R, Rollnick S 1991 Motivational interviewing: preparing people to change addictive behavior. Guilford Press, New York

Sesney J W, Kreher N E, Hickner J M, Webb S 1997 Smoking cessation interventions in rural family practices: An UPRNet study. Journal of Family Practice 44:578–585

7

Training health professionals

Training people to use this approach is, in essence, an intervention to encourage behavior change. There is very little said about patient behavior change in the rest of this book that cannot be applied to practitioners. This chapter contains some hints based on our own experiences of training practitioners to use this method. It describes the issues to consider in making your decisions about what to teach and how best to do so.

GIVE US THE MAGIC BULLET

The training of practitioners is sometimes viewed as an inconvenient byproduct of a more worthy endeavor: getting the patients to change. All one needs, it is believed, is a workshop for the practitioners to 'get them skilled up' and then we can get the patients on the right road. How one wishes it was as simple as that. As a trainer one cannot escape this oversimplified view of skill acquisition, which is most prevalent in commissioning and research communities. Fortunately, the practitioners one trains usually know better; that their consulting styles, however flexible they might be, do not change overnight. Training is not a matter of replacing one bag of tools with another, but of subtle alterations to a repertoire which needs gradual and ongoing fine tuning to meet the needs of the shifting and sensitive world of behavior change. Sustained change will not be achieved by a dose of anything, be it a workshop or a spectacularly good consultation. Knowledge of this reality is the most important training guideline. It calls for humility, sensitivity to trainees' clinical reality and a keen eye on the horizon. If you present trainees with an oversimplified blueprint, the exercise is probably dead before it starts. On the other hand, if you wallow with them in the endless complexity of human interaction about behavior change, the outcome will be the same. The answer lies in finding a balance between the two, by providing some structure for discussion and skills acquisition and a solid injection of real-world clinical problems. How to achieve this is the subject of this chapter.

CONTEXT, LANGUAGE AND THE MEETING OF CULTURES

This method, with its underlying values and terms, is not always congruent with the clinical environment one encounters. For example, we have worked on the introduction of this patient-centered method into an emergency room setting, where all the emphasis is understandably on doing things to patients, on fixing them up. The problem was, staff were frustrated by the number of times they saw the same patients, returning time and again with the violent consequences of behavioral problems like drug and alcohol misuse. They wanted to find ways of encouraging patients to seek counseling (Bernstein et al 1997). Another striking example was the need of a military organization to find new ways of talking to people who fail their annual fitness test. Training, like traveling, is thus an adventure in meeting new ways of thinking and talking.

The solution, we believe, is not to try and change the value base of the practitioners who work in these settings, but to work with their language and values to accommodate the kind of methods we believe might be of use to them. This often means avoiding the use of jargon as much as possible, and listening carefully to how they describe their everyday work problems. It should then be possible to design training that is congruent with their needs. Our military colleagues, for example, very much liked the metaphor of a toolbox, because it was compatible with so much of their everyday work. The toolbox contained tools which were used to encourage choice and decision making in their clients. On the other hand, the emergency room team, used as they were to calming the tempers of distressed, intoxicated and sometimes violent patients, preferred to describe their behavior change work as a brief negotiated interview, in which a rather rushed but respectful attempt was made to encourage referral to counseling.

PLANNING

What is your brief?

Your trainees want to learn how to motivate patients to change their behavior. You, in turn, want to motivate them to consider changing their behavior in their consultations. You need, therefore, to understand the training situation from their point of view. Consider asking yourself the following questions as you plan.

Who asked you to do the training and why?

- What is the problem to which they think your training might be the solution?
- What is the relationship between the person who set up the training and the trainees?
- Will the trainees have been 'sent' on the course?

- Is the course a hoop through which trainees have to jump in order to achieve something else?

In planning a workshop it is important to understand, as well as possible, the motives of all concerned. People organize and fund such events for a range of reasons and these may affect the process. Here are two examples of scenarios we have encountered:

1. A health organization commissioned compulsory training in behavior change for nurses in a family practice setting. The training was intended to help ensure the quality of health promotion work. However, it could have been seen by some of the health practitioners as an unwanted hoop through which they had to jump before getting funding. It was, for some, part of a bureaucratic structure rather than a valued opportunity for professional development.
2. A pharmaceutical firm commissioned training on behavior change to help practitioners to improve patient compliance in using prophylactic medication. The apparent interests of patients, health professionals and the pharmaceutical firm were found to be similar. Patients do not want to be given drugs they have no wish to take and the health professionals are not comfortable in a situation in which they experience repeated failure in getting patients to do what they think is good for them. Neither does it enhance the reputation of the drugs in question if they are given to patients who do not want them, do not take them properly and thus do not show any improvement in their health. Ensuring that patients get only the medication they are willing to take was of interest to both commissioners of the training and the trainees, and was compatible with the spirit of patient empowerment.

Who are the prospective trainees?

Whether or not you already know the group, it is worth enquiring into contextual matters in some depth before you start.

- What is in it for them to learn this approach?
- What do the trainees already know? For example, can you assume they are familiar with listening skills and have a commitment to a patient-centered approach?
- How will you check their existing knowledge and skills so as not to waste time going over old ground?
- What communication problems arise in their everyday work with patients?
- What might their hopes and fears be about you and the training?
- How ready do you think they might be to adopt a new style of intervention?

What impact might all this have on the trainees' attitude to the training? Can you identify or predict any specific areas of reluctance or resistance? If so, how can you apply some of the principles of the method itself to addressing them?

Other learning opportunities

Workshops and seminars are only part of the process of practitioners assimilating new ways of working. To make the most of your teaching opportunity, be aware of and take advantage of the other ways your trainees might learn this approach.

- How else will they be able to learn?
- Will the trainees expect or be able to read around the topic before or after the training event?
- Will they have opportunities for supervised practice? If so, are there any ways you can help them and their supervisors to structure the supervision so as to promote skills development?
- Is follow-up training planned? If so, how can you and they best use this and the intervening weeks?

Your goals

It is commonly believed that the purpose of training is to enhance *skills* (confidence). However, in teaching this approach there is an equally relevant task: helping practitioners to value this patient-centered approach (importance). Thus, the concepts of confidence and importance can be useful guides for training practitioners. A purely skills-based workshop might meet with resistance because, for some of the practitioners, there is a more fundamental problem: they do not see the value of the method in the first place. Enhancing this perception of value might require a focus on their *knowledge* and relevant scientific evidence, and their *attitudes* towards behavior change consultations. They might not want, for example, to practice skills, but might value looking at demonstrations or role-playing a patient, and so on. The more you know about your trainees the easier it will be to decide what the goals of the workshop should be.

What can you realistically achieve with this particular group?

- How familiar and comfortable are they with a patient-centered approach and the concept of client responsibility?
- Does the rest of their professional practice foster the attitudes compatible with the spirit of the method? (Or are they more accustomed to being emphatic than empathic?)

- Will you have *time* to teach the techniques well? Is there any risk that in trying to teach the techniques too quickly you will raise trainees' awareness of what they cannot do, without enabling competence?

Some of the following behavioral objectives for a session might be selected by the trainer. By the end of the workshop or educational program, trainees will be able to:

- describe a model for understanding changing lifestyle behaviors
- raise the issue of lifestyle change with a patient in a way that does not elicit resistance
- use an agenda-setting strategy to help a patient decide what changes he or she might talk about
- use the model and associated visual aids to assess a patient's feelings about change (readiness, importance and confidence)
- assist a patient in exploring the importance of a particular behavior change and the confidence to achieve it
- use a range of active listening skills to enable a patient to clarify his or her own feelings about lifestyle change
- conduct a consultation in such a way as to leave the responsibility for change, and the right to decide whether or not to change, clearly with the patient
- give accurate and appropriate information about lifestyle and health in a neutral way and enable the patient to interpret the implications for his or her own situation
- describe how they handle their own frustrations when working with patients who do not, at present, want to change; and how they avoid attempting to impose their own timetable for change upon the patient
- describe an overview of the method's tasks and strategies
- use a menu of strategies for guiding the consultation.

Which strategies to teach?

The preceding chapters suggest a wide range of strategies that can be used by health professionals. It will rarely be appropriate to teach them all in a single workshop but it can be difficult to decide what to include and what to omit. Tober (1993) in a discussion of social work training, describes the *need to know principle* and the importance of *solving problems, not creating problems*. The content of a workshop needs to relate as closely as possible to the participants' everyday practice. Busy professionals learn, not just out of academic interest but in the hope that they will become better able to help their clients or patients and/or make their own working lives easier. They do not want to be overwhelmed by interesting but irrelevant ideas or by descriptions of interventions that they do not have the time or facilities to put into practice. A clear understanding of trainees' occupational remit helps the trainer to identify which aspects of the method will be of most value. If one has time, the ideal format is to help trainees select which strategies best suit their needs. They construct their own menu of strategies which suits their work setting. Here are a number of examples we have encountered:

- Nurses running a smoking clinic will be less concerned than most with *raising the issue*. They will not need to learn how to *set an agenda* by choosing between *multiple behaviors*. Their remit is clear and their patients know what the agenda is when they accept the appointment. Strategies for assessing importance and confidence will, however, be very useful in planning their work with particular patients.
- Family doctors running a 5- to 10-minute appointment system will need to learn the strategies that can be accomplished in a minute or two. To teach them to use strategies such as *A Typical Day* will, in many cases, present them with time-management difficulties. *Agenda setting* can be very useful for starting a consultation about behavior change, and *scaling questions* will help them to make quick assessments within their time constraints, thus solving rather than creating problems for them.
- Dieticians who see their patients for longer appointments may value a strategy such as *A Typical Day* due to the complex way in which eating is woven into everyday activities. They should have the time to use it. They might also find the *stress bucket* a useful way of seeing where comfort eating fits into everyday life.

Training time

In a course of two days or more, it may be possible to achieve all of the above objectives. For a short course it will be necessary to prioritize. Trainers usually feel that they are not given enough time to teach their material thoroughly, whatever the topic. In some educational settings, for example qualifying training for health professionals, the actual contact time that trainers have with students is only intended to be a small part of the learning time. Students are expected to do a considerable amount of reading to supplement lectures and seminars. However, in postgraduate training and on in-service courses there is sometimes an expectation that almost all of the learning will take place in the time allocated to the training session itself. If a single lecture only is available, the trainer can expect to be able to tell trainees *about* the method, explaining the spirit and the tasks and giving examples of strategies. It will be up to each individual to teach him- or herself how to put it into practice through experimenting with colleagues and patients. A 2- or 3-day workshop will enable its trainees to absorb the spirit thoroughly and become reasonably comfortable with performing the tasks, practicing some of the strategies and using the visual aids.

How much time trainees need will, of course, depend to some extent on what they already know and can do. It is much easier and quicker to teach this method to trainees with a background in patient-centered consulting skills. The spirit of the method will be familiar to them and they will already have some ability to use listening skills.

It is our experience as trainers that the spirit is more important than the techniques. Practitioners with good basic consultation skills, if they fully grasp and embrace the spirit of negotiation, will be able to work out some strategies and techniques for themselves. Practitioners who learn some techniques but have not fully assimilated the spirit will not be able to use those techniques properly and will not experience a real change in the process of their consultations.

Similarly, as regards the visual aids and tools, these are very tangible and attractive to practitioners. They can *enhance* the basic approach of the method, but are not the method itself. In a short session it can be tempting to focus disproportionately on such tangible items and miss out on the underlying theory and spirit that is the crucial underpinning to their use.

Once you are clear what you are trying to achieve it will be easier to identify the best training methods.

DELIVERING TRAINING

Do you practice what you preach and provide a role model for encouraging behavior change? Ask yourself the following with regard to your training methods.

- Are your training methods congruent with the principles of negotiating behavior change?
- How can you provide a clear structure whilst leaving responsibility for learning with the trainees?
- How can you best avoid an evangelical approach which might elicit resistance?
- How can you provide an opportunity for trainees to consider, for themselves, the *importance* of adopting a new approach to their consultations?
- How can you help trainees develop *confidence* in their new skills? What are the best ways to organize demonstrations and practice sessions in order to empower them (rather than merely show up their skill deficits)?
- How can you best help trainees transfer existing skills from other areas of their work to enhance their consultations about behavior change?
- How are you going to monitor and reduce resistance during the course of the training?

Implications of the size of the group

As all experienced trainers will know, the size of the group will be a major factor affecting the extent to which trainees participate in discussion. As the spirit of the method is so important, it is necessary to aim for an environment in which all participants (not just the most vocal) can talk through their questions, reservations and ambivalence about this way of working. Once a group goes above 20 in size it is difficult to seat everyone in a single circle or horseshoe. This, in itself, affects the dynamics, and the shyer or more reserved trainees become reluctant to speak out. Where large groups cannot be avoided, doing some of the work in small groups will, to some extent, overcome the problem, especially if there is more than one trainer to help monitor and facilitate discussions.

The spirit of the training

Chapter 2 says patients have freedom of choice: it is not appropriate to force our views upon them and the practitioner's role is to help patients to make decisions within their own frame of reference. It also refers to the importance of working in a way that is congruent with each patient's level of readiness to change. These principles can be applied very effectively to training as well as to consultations. People attend training for a wide variety of reasons. Rarely do they arrive determined to soak up every word the trainer says so that they can go away and change their practice accordingly. Often they arrive a little suspicious or cynical. They expect to be bored or told things they already know. Sometimes they are anxious that they will be exposed as poor practitioners or found to be less well informed than others in the group. These attitudes affect the process: the wise trainer will set up exercises that elicit expressions of these attitudes and give the unsure plenty of opportunity to contemplate. This book emphasizes that people need time to think about change and to consider its importance and their confidence to take action. There are obvious parallels between the work with patients and the process of training people to do it.

The implication of all this, applied to training, is that a lecture on how students ought to run their consultations, with exhortations to go away and practice differently is, in its very process and style, undermining the principles that the lecturer is trying to convey. However charismatic the presentation, such a lecture is unlikely to have the desired effect on all trainees. The alternative is to present ideas and then create opportunities for trainees to consider their own ambivalence about them. Trainees can be encouraged to discuss whether or not they consider an idea valid or useful and whether they can imagine themselves changing their practice to incorporate the method.

In trying to assimilate new ideas, people often look for the parts with which they disagree and argue about them. The trainer, in handling such 'questions' or confrontations may at first feel threatened and tempted to act defensively. In fact, he or she has been presented with the ideal opportunity to model how to relate to someone who is unsure about change. An appropriate response is to summarize the disagreements or concerns, exchange information, and clarify any points of confusion. Finally the trainee can be left to reflect on whether to explore further how to use the method, without precipitating any confrontation during the course of the workshop.

So, the general approach to the training needs to be compatible with the principles you are trying to teach. If at any point the training seems to be going badly and you are encountering resistance, the principles of the method itself will help you to identify the problem and how to proceed. One creative way of linking the two is to ask the trainees, part way through the course, to rate the method. They can be asked to assess its *importance* to their work and their *confidence* in using it. As in the strategy outlined in Chapter 4, 1–10 scaling questions can be used for this purpose. You can then ask what it would take to move them along a little and tailor the next section of the workshop accordingly.

Using yourself to best advantage

Trainees demand a great deal from their trainers. Reflecting on your own talents and experiences will help you to continually improve.

- How are you going to make the most of your own strengths and overcome any weaknesses as a trainer?
- Are you competent at negotiating behavior change? If you are a skilled practitioner, how can you help your trainees to benefit from your skills? If not, how can you accommodate your trainees' requests for examples or demonstrations of techniques?
- Are you familiar with the academic and research base for this type of approach to behavior change consultations? How will you ensure that trainees get as much information about this as is useful to them without overloading them?
- Will your professional or academic background make you immediately credible and trustworthy to this particular group of trainees and, if so, how will you make the best of this? If not, how will you establish rapport with them at an early stage?

Frequently we have found that the best way to illustrate a particular point is to demonstrate it, using a co-trainer or trainee as 'patient'. This points to a necessity for the trainer to be fluent in using the method so as to be able to selectively demonstrate key strategies or tasks. Sometimes demonstrations go wrong and the trainer needs to be both confident and humble enough to admit mistakes and to turn such situations into useful learning experiences for everyone. Trainees will ideally learn to adapt the method to suit their own styles of working while keeping the spirit and principles intact. Highly skilled and charismatic trainers need to be careful not to imply that trainees should aim to copy the trainer's style and not to intimidate trainees through giving too many polished performances.

WAYS TO GET THE MESSAGE ACROSS

The discussion above regarding the spirit of training suggests the need for participatory teaching methods. The trainer's role is to set up opportunities for trainees to explore issues and adapt strategies to their own situations. A training program as such is not given here. As already discussed, the content of such a program would need to be designed around the needs of each particular group. A progression from exploration of the spirit and principles on to description and demonstration of the method, followed by practice opportunities, generally works well. Below is a selection of training methods that we have found useful in teaching this approach. Trainers may wish to add some of these to their own repertoire of training exercises or adapt them as appropriate. The suggestions below relate to:

- beginning a workshop
- illustrating the spirit
- illustrating the method or strategies within it
- structuring opportunities for practice
- bringing a workshop to a close.

Beginning a workshop

In introducing any workshop on this method, the priority will be to create an appropriate climate in the group. Trainees will need to feel able to wonder aloud about the spirit of the method and the implications of using it in practice. They will need to be able to try out new intervention skills without being overwhelmingly afraid of looking foolish, and to challenge some of their own beliefs or assumptions. Trainers will have their own favorite exercises for climate building and may consider including the following:

- working in small groups discussing trainees' hopes and fears about the workshop and the skills and qualities they bring to it
- trainees introducing themselves in a way that brings in some non-threatening personal disclosure (e.g. hobbies, unusual claims to fame, origins of their names),
- setting ground rules for the workshop that include willingness to take some risks, to challenge and to be challenged, and to maintain appropriate confidentiality boundaries.

If trainees are not accustomed to participative skills training then it will be necessary to discuss the following:

- participation is encouraged, but if anyone, for any reason, wishes to drop out of a specific exercise they can 'pass' on it
- the pace, and to a certain extent the content, of the workshop can and will be adapted as it goes along to better meet emerging trainee need.

Agreement on key issues (in effect making a contract between trainer and trainees) at the beginning can make it easier to deal with any difficulties later.

Illustrating the spirit

Chapter 3 contains a list of dangerous assumptions. We have found that discussion of these facilitates trainees to become accustomed to the spirit of negotiation. It brings out, at an early stage, in a fairly specific way, any resistance they have to working in this way.

To do this, go through the dangerous assumptions on a slide or transparency, clarifying what each means and describing briefly any ways in which it might sometimes obstruct the process of negotiating lifestyle change. Do not discuss the assumptions at this stage. This might take 10 minutes. Split trainees into groups (6–8 individuals is a good size) and give them all paper copies of the list of dangerous assumptions. Instruct each group to pick out any of the statements that they find particularly interesting or challenging and discuss them. Allow about 30 minutes for this. Ask each group to feed back one important point, briefly, to a plenary session.

Trainees will thus sometimes raise issues in which they disagree with the trainer's views. The trainer (remembering the task of understanding ambivalence), clarifies their views if necessary but resists the temptation to resolve the ambivalence or tell the group members how they should feel. The discussion will highlight the role that values play in behavior change consultations. The ethical issues and their practical implications are discussed in detail in Chapter 2.

For some trainees this exercise will enable them to see that this method is for them: it is compatible with their beliefs about their work. For others it will begin a process of contemplating another way of looking at things. This process cannot successfully be hurried.

Illustrating the method

'A picture paints a thousand words' and a demonstration can, on a good day, explain more than a lecture ever can. It may illustrate a particular strategy or show, in conjunction with the overview diagram, how all the elements fit together. Trainees often comment after seeing a demonstration that it has helped them to realize that the method is not a mechanistic process. They can see that when strategies are selected and chosen in the right spirit the consultation flows and is responsive to patient need. Some advantages of demonstrating the method are:

- it is a vivid way of showing exactly what you mean
- it demonstrates that the trainer actually has real clinical skills and is not afraid to put them on the line to be criticized by the group
- it breaks up a 'chalk-and-talk' presentation and regains participants' interest
- it roots theory in practice.

One disadvantage is:

- if it is done *very* well, less confident trainees can feel de-skilled, feeling that they have been set a goal that is, for them, unrealistic.

Some ways that it can go wrong are:

- there is not enough time left afterwards for analysis and discussion, so that the demonstration has good entertainment value but trainees do not translate what they have seen into what they themselves could do
- a 'patient' for the role-play is drawn from the 'audience'. A very compliant, eager-to-please trainee plays a patient who is so ready to change that the trainer cannot demonstrate the negotiation process at all
- a 'patient' for the role-play is drawn from the 'audience'. A trainee volunteers and plays a patient who has a range of overwhelming problems. It eventually becomes clear that negotiation of lifestyle change is way down the list of help needed and crisis intervention is what is required. (Often, in these circumstances the volunteer afterwards sheepishly admits that he or she volunteered to play that particular patient because they had been struggling to help such a patient for ages and thought they might 'pick up a few tips' from the trainer).

So what does this teach us? Role-play demonstrations need to be set up very carefully in order to show what you actually want to demonstrate. If there is the luxury of a second trainer, it might be better to use him or her as the patient (although this lays you open to the charge of having 'rigged' it so it will go well). Allow at least as much time for discussion as the role-play itself takes and be generous in drawing attention to any less than perfect interventions by the 'health professional'. Frequently such mistakes will help illustrate key learning points and the process will also encourage trainees to take risks later if asked to do role-plays themselves.

An alternative to live demonstration is to show a video. There are two types of video used to illustrate consultation approaches: stand-alone teaching materials and recordings of real or role-played consultations illustrating key points.

Stand-alone videos usually contain a short lecture as well as demonstrations and illustrations. They can be useful to supplement a workshop as trainees can watch them at home as preparation or revision. There are problems in using them as part of a workshop. Watching videos tends to be a passive rather than an active process. Sitting trainees in front of a screen for long periods can undo the work done to build an active, participative climate.

Trainers who have access to stand-alone videos that they feel present the issues better than they could do it 'live' can avoid this problem to some extent. The film can be shown in small sections, introducing discussion or practice exercises between the sections.

Videos of consultations to illustrate key points can be helpful. They avoid some of the disadvantages and risks of live demonstrations as described above. As with a live demonstration, time for analysis and discussion afterwards is important.

One way of showing this approach clearly is to demonstrate how it differs (as an intervention and in terms of the patients' responses) from other common ways of approaching behavior change. Trainees can learn either by watching or by doing it themselves, how a few minutes of confrontation and advice-giving differs from an empathic, patient-centered exploration of the issues. If trainees are to do this themselves it needs to be clearly thought out and clear instructions given, ideally in a handout sheet. As in the role-play practice discussed below, trainees may either role-play patients for this or use their own material.

Structuring opportunities for practice

'Everyone hates role-play' but 'practice makes perfect'. Before refining their skills through their work with patients, trainees do need to learn the basics by practicing on each other. The challenge for the trainer is to find the best way to set up such an exercise. There are several different ways of organizing role-play practice:

- pairs of trainees can work without being observed
- in trios they can take it in turns to watch and give feedback to each other
- a pair can perform in front of a group in a 'fishbowl' situation
- role-play can be video-recorded for criticizing afterwards either in the group or in a one-to-one situation.

Practicing without feedback from one or more observers can limit skills development but having one's attempts to practice new skills observed by a peer provokes anxiety. A little anxiety helps people to learn, but too much inhibits the process.

One way of providing valuable role-play practice without provoking excessive anxiety is to set it up not as a performance but as an experiment.

One person role-plays a client, the second experiments with negotiating behavior change and the third acts as consultant. At any time the experimenter can call 'time-out' from the role-play. They can then talk through with the consultant any difficulties that are arising, or just allow themselves time to think what to ask or say next and how best to phrase it. Similarly, at any time the consultant can indicate to the experimenter, by a tap on the shoulder, that she or he has an observation or suggestion to make. The experimenter can choose whether to ignore it for now and continue, or whether to call time-out and hear what the consultant has to say.

We have found that this way of conducting a role-play enables people to give themselves permission to take risks and try out new techniques. The more traditional method of using a third person as an observer tends to encourage people to put on their best performance, which usually means using tried and tested techniques with which they feel confident. The observer then empathizes with their anxiety (especially if it is their turn next) and gives very positive feedback, resulting in everybody confirming the way they all worked before the course began.

Role-play can be an opportunity for practicing the underpinning listening skills and the strategies specific to this method. It can be set up so that trainees work on a particular chosen strategy or skill. Alternatively it can be left open for them to respond to the issues that arise in the role-play consultation.

It can be empowering to invite trainees, before taking their turn at practicing, to decide on their own individual specific behavior change objective for the role-play. The consultant can then be asked specifically to help in working towards this. For example, one trainee might choose to try to understand a patient's ambivalence without getting into an argument about why he or she should change. Another might experiment with allowing more silences to give the patient time to think. Yet another might aim to check what the patient already knows before rushing in to tell him or her a heap of facts. Choosing one key behavior to change both makes the task manageable and enables trainees to evaluate their own progress.

There are advantages in preparing role-play case studies for people. These can be designed to meet the needs of the moment. The trainer can set up the role-play to require *raising the issue*. Alternatively, a situation can be presented where the issue is already on the agenda and the task is to assess readiness to change. Some of the scenarios given in Chapter 6 could form the basis for such pre-prepared case studies. Alternatives are to get people to role-play real patients that they have seen recently or to use real issues and material from their own lives.

It is important to brief trainees carefully about selecting their own material to bring to an exercise. The issue needs to be important enough to be worth talking about but not a major life crisis. Trainees need to be clearly reminded that the exercise is not intended as therapy for them but is a vehicle for learning about intervention skills. Occasionally someone will begin talking about a behavior change issue and will discover after a few minutes that it is more emotionally laden than they had realized. The trainer needs to be sensitive to this and be able to give the trainee clear permission to stop the exercise and take care of his or her own needs before returning to the workshop. However, the advantage of trainees using their own material is that they experience more sharply their own resistance to confrontation and their more positive response to other approaches.

Bringing a workshop to a close

If it has not already arisen in discussion (which it may well have done), it is worth spending some time considering the big question: how does all this relate to my everyday work? This helps trainees to bridge the gap between an intensive training experience and everyday practice. It is also useful before closing a workshop to help trainees to link the experience with other learning opportunities. They can be asked to rate their own commitment to learning to use the method and their confidence in doing so, and to identify the next step.

A closing round of 'one helpful thing I have learned from today and one thing I intend to do differently over the next few weeks' can be useful in enabling people to clarify their achievements. This can foster the necessary confidence.

EVALUATION

Once you are clear what you want to teach and how, you can begin to see how you might evaluate your training. Evaluation can be in terms of outcome: did the workshop achieve what it set out to do? and process: did it achieve the outcome in an appropriate way?

Evaluation by outcome is considerably easier if there are clear objectives at the beginning. An evaluation form can then solicit trainees' views about whether the course met its objectives. Trainers' own observations of contributions to discussions and practice sessions will be another source of data about outcome. As with consultations, if the person decides not to change, the intervention was not a failure. The workshop will be an opportunity for trainees to learn how to do something and decide whether to do it or not. We know we cannot make people change so it is inappropriate to judge our own performance by whether they do or not. Evaluation of the process will include consideration of whether

- the training methods chosen facilitated the learning process
- all the items of content were given an appropriate amount of attention

- the process demonstrated an appropriate value base, that is, respect for trainees, trainee-centered learning and an anti-discriminatory approach.

Ideally evaluation will include an assessment of the trainees before the training. What do they already know? What can they do? What do they want? An assessment of the *process* needs to take place soon after the workshop itself and an assessment of *outcome* in practice is most realistic some weeks after the training.

CONCLUSION

Training on this method needs to be based on the principles of the method itself. This includes respect for the trainees' right to make their own decisions about whether to change and use the method. It also includes an acknowledgement that it may take more than one training session for someone to gain the motivation and the confidence to put a new way of working into practice. (Handouts and other written material are useful for providing reference for people who come back to these ideas some time after the course.) The spirit of negotiation is very important and should not be neglected, even in a short session. Participative training methods undoubtedly make it easier to work at the trainees' own pace and enable them to explore fully the issues that are important for them.

REFERENCES

Bernstein E, Bernstein J, Levenson S 1997 Project Assert: an ed-based intervention to increase access to primary care preventive services and the substance abuse treatment system. Annals of Emergency Medicine 30:181–189
Tober G 1993 A strategy for social work training. In: Harrison L (ed) Substance misuse: designing social work training. Central Council for Education and Training in Social Work and University of Hull.

8

Broader horizons

In aiming to be practical in earlier chapters, we put to one side a number of clinical, ethical and theoretical issues. Sometimes they took the form of assumptions that we were making, which felt fragile to say the least (e.g. behavior change is a good idea for all). At other points we oversimplified in order to keep to task. In this chapter we will free ourselves from the need to be pragmatic, and discuss issues which illustrate that health behavior change is a fertile ground for research, further clinical innovation and debate.

FROM THE CONCEPTUAL WORLD TO CLINICAL PRACTICE

Readiness, importance and confidence revisited

In Chapter 2 we described readiness as a relatively more global state of mind, influenced to a large extent by perceived importance and perceived confidence (see Figure 2.3, p. 22). Practitioners might find it helpful to think of the relationship between the three concepts in the manner illustrated in Figure 8.1 below. For example, if individuals A and B were excessive drinkers, they might both feel not ready to change, but for completely different reasons. Drinker A might feel that it is very important to change, perhaps because of a physical illness, but feel very pessimistic about his or her ability to succeed. In contrast, drinker B might feel confident about succeeding with reduced consumption, were he to try, but does not feel it is important to do this at the present time. Obviously, drinker C has high levels of both importance and confidence and is therefore much more ready to change than the other two.

Our goal here is to provide practitioners with a conceptual aid for guiding conversations about change, not to construct a comprehensive model of behavior change. In the interests of science, it is tempting to make Figure 8.1 much more complicated. Where, for example, are a wide range of contextual factors represented? In making decisions to change a specific behavior, patients have to take into account what will happen to their moods, other behaviors and other people. Everyday pressures, problems and pleasures do not disappear or remain static when we make changes in a particular behavior. However, in the consulting room, the practitioner does not

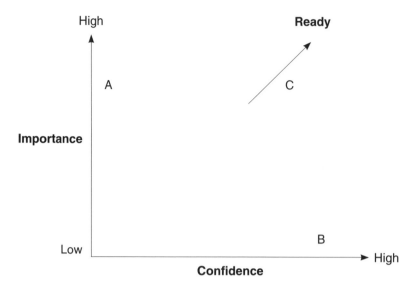

Figure 8.1 Readiness, importance and confidence: a practitioner's guide.

experience these contextual forces as separate from feelings about importance, confidence and readiness. In fact, conversations about importance, confidence and readiness usually form the channels through which contextual forces are expressed: they become the keys to unlocking the personal context in which the behavior occurs. For example, ask a patient about importance and the conversation might focus on the specific behavior or it might turn to talk about personal values, other priorities, or the effect of change on something else like stress levels, a close relationship, and so on. Talk about confidence to achieve change and contextual matters will come tumbling down into the consulting room. Suddenly, for example, loneliness might emerge as a bigger priority than behavior change. Similarly, talk about readiness, particularly if the patient is close to decision making, and the discussion will turn to matters of timing and other priorities. The value of these concepts lies precisely in the opportunity they provide to talk about the context in which the behavior in question occurs.

One clear limitation of Figure 8.1 and our discussion of it is that, like most models of behavior change in health psychology, the focus is upon a single behavior only. The subtle interrelationships between health behaviors, which are the daily currency of talk in the consulting room, are thus not taken into account. A change in one behavior often affects others. Although we have tried to capture these challenges in a practical way, with the use of an agenda-setting strategy for dealing with multiple behaviors in Chapter 3, we have not taken the theoretical leap and considered how readiness, importance and confidence change across different behaviors in different circumstances. Neither have we considered in sufficient detail what happens when the readiness of the practitioner to meet patient requests is challenged (see this chapter p. 199 and Chapter 6 pp. 156–167).

Building a bridge between theory and everyday practice is an uncomfortable journey, in which theoreticians will justifiably be concerned about oversimplification and practitioners will react against jargon and what they see as needless complexity. The stages of change model, which we turn to next, has been useful precisely because it crosses this divide with conceptual clarity and a good dose of common sense.

Readiness and stages of change: some unresolved issues

For some years now, the stages of change framework has stimulated research and clinical development across a wide range of fields. One of us recently received a request to discuss its application to obese household pets! Reviews and critiques can be found in Miller & Heather (1998) and Bandura (1995). Of particular interest are issues which revolve around the use of the stages of change model by practitioners to provide the rationale for intervention. The problem here is that making judgments about readiness, particularly if one is wedded to using stage labels, can be complex and have unfortunate, sometimes unintended, consequences. At best, these judgments are the outcome of genuine consensus between practitioner and patient. At worst, they can be oversimplified and driven by the prejudices of the practitioner. Four of the most commonly encountered difficulties are discussed below.

Let's not waste time on the precontemplators

Precontemplation, as noted in Chapter 2, is the first stage of change in the model developed by Prochaska & DiClemente (1983). We often hear the following sentiment expressed by practitioners: '*If they are obviously not ready to change, leave them alone: concentrate your energies on those who are more ready to change*'. This interpretation of the stages of change model, as Ashworth (1997) has noted, can serve as a valuable stress reduction strategy: '… the model can provide a rationale for staff to give up struggling with those who are reluctant to change' (Ashworth 1997, p. 167). In other words, one can avoid unnecessary conflict by ignoring the precontemplators. This approach probably occurs quite naturally in everyday practice. For example, some American research shows that precontemplators are least likely to receive an intervention about smoking from their primary care physicians (Sesney et al 1997).

One can understand a busy practitioner, faced by a daily flood of faces, making this kind of decision on an individual basis about where to invest one's energy. Many a wise practitioner decides to leave an issue to one side, in the hope of strengthening the relationship so that it can be tackled at a later date. However, it is one thing to make delicate decisions under time pressure, with the patient's interests firmly in mind; it is another altogether to adhere to a *general guideline* which results in no discussion with precontemplators.

This practice is certainly not recommended in any of the writing of Prochaska, DiClemente and colleagues. In fact, they even talk of the need for a 'paradigm' shift away from services which focus only on those who are ready to change (DiClemente & Prochaska 1998). The main problem with neglecting to intervene with precontemplators is that we label patients with a stage-linked identity, almost like a trait, when we know their expressed feelings about change are context bound and changeable. We then descend into dichotomous thinking, e.g. 'people are either motivated or not', and lose one of the most appealing features of the stages of change model, namely that practitioners need to be responsive to the wide range of patient views and feelings about change. It then becomes fairly easy to justify not working with the 'unmotivated'. This is what happened in the specialist addictions field for many decades: treatment was only geared around those who were really ready to change (a small minority). Patients expressing ambivalence were labeled as unmotivated, not amenable to help from an action-oriented treatment system. The possibility of finding ways of talking to less ready sufferers remained buried beneath a sea of dogma (see Davies 1979, 1981; Miller & Rollnick 1991).

Patients labeled as precontemplators are quite diverse, an observation which led DiClemente (1991) to distinguish between reluctant, rebellious, resigned and rationalizing individuals. There might be ways of talking to such people without reinforcing resistance and disagreement. Indeed, we believe that a sensitive assessment of readiness, importance and confidence often facilitates achieving this goal. Interviews conducted among family practitioners who were trained to use this strategy reported positive experiences of using it, and this included talking about change among smokers who were far from ready to take action (Rollnick et al 1997a). Precontemplators might be more open to change than we think, a view supported by some of our recent research: heavy drinkers engaged in a health promotion discussion who were less ready to change fared better when faced with brief motivational interviewing than with a skills-based intervention (Heather et al 1996). Along similar lines, we were surprised to find that smokers identified by practitioners as precontemplators responded better to intervention based on the assessment of importance and confidence than to simple advice-giving (Butler et al, in press). DiClemente & Prochaska (1998) also report a number of studies in which it proved possible to improve retention rates among smoking precontemplators. To write off precontemplators as not likely to benefit from an intervention is premature.

Readiness to do what?

Stage labels are frequently used by practitioners and researchers without clear reference to exactly what the behavior change in question is. This gives rise to confusion and oversimplification.

Some behavior changes seem more complex than others. Stopping smoking is a relatively simple example, where a consultation often involves a single event: quitting. Making a judgment about readiness can be fairly straightforward. In contrast, with dietary changes for example, there is usually not one but a range of changes to consider. These could involve adjustments, reductions, omissions or new additions to eating behavior, or perhaps a combination of these strategies. Readiness to make these changes will vary. I might be very ready to eat more fruit, definitely not ready to eat less chocolate, and confused about the whole issue of reducing red meat intake. How will a practitioner judge my readiness to make dietary change?

The exact words the practitioner uses are also important. Ask a heavy drinker how ready she feels about the following changes and you might emerge with different judgments about readiness: *How ready are you to talk about your drinking?; … to think about changing your drinking habits?; … to reduce your drinking on weekends?; … to stop drinking for ever?*

Many patients we talk to are not only considering changes in a specific behavior like eating, smoking or drinking, but in other aspects of their lives as well. Readiness to change will vary across all of these potential changes, not just in the problem behavior. Ask the above heavy drinker about her life as a whole, and you will emerge with different judgments about readiness. Thus, she might be a precontemplator in relation to complete abstinence (often the practitioner's main priority), a contemplator about reduced alcohol intake, in the preparation stage about eating healthier foods and in the action stage about ensuring that her children are better cared for.

Sometimes, particularly in chronic disease clinics, change or improvement is not a realistic goal for the patients. Staying the same, or not getting worse, is what is talked about in consultations. A readiness assessment in these circumstances needs to be adjusted accordingly.

These challenges are not insurmountable in the consulting room. Knowing which kind of question to ask about readiness (or importance and confidence) requires skillful observation, judgment, a good sense of timing, and careful listening. It seems clear, however, that judgments about readiness should be *specific* to a particular change. These observations do not undermine the validity of the concept of readiness or the stages of change model. They do, however, caution against the oversimplified use of judgments of readiness, particularly when an individual is assigned to a stage that hangs over him like a flag which determines how he is to be approached by a practitioner. For example, to label the above woman in trouble with alcohol as a precontemplator says only a little about her, and quite a lot about the priorities and prejudices of the practitioner. Treatment systems or guidelines for practitioners geared around stage labels could thus carry a serious risk of oversimplification. We turn now to what is probably the most common example of this kind of thinking.

The contemplators need 'motivational' help; those more ready need a more practical intervention

This an example of matching talk, about how to match an intervention to the stage of change of the individual. Practitioners and trainers, ourselves included, have presented this example of matching as one of the key messages of the stages of change model: contemplators need help to weigh up the pros and cons of change (often called a *motivational intervention*), while those in the preparation stage need help with practical matters: techniques and strategies for improving confidence to cope with behavior change (*skills-based intervention*). Clinical guidelines have been based on this notion (e.g. Annis et al 1996), and one recent line of research into matching has investigated this hypothesis carefully (Heather et al 1996, Project MATCH Research Group 1997).

There seems to be some validity to this particular way of matching interventions to stages. Progression through stages does involve a shift in people's perceptions of the costs and benefits of change (Velicer et al 1985, Prochaska 1994, Prochaska et al 1994), and less ready smokers and heavy drinkers do seem to respond better to a less action-oriented discussion of change (Heather et al 1996, Butler et al, in press, Project MATCH Research Group 1997). However, these research findings should not be overstated, because the effects observed are not uniformly strong. Moreover, it has not emerged that those who are *more ready* to change respond better to a skills-based approach, despite the observation that self-efficacy, according to Prochaska & DiClemente (1998), is more important during the later stages of change.

There is a strong possibility that we have oversimplified the needs of people in different stages of change. Concerns about importance (pros and cons) are not necessarily restricted to the contemplation stage but can emerge in the preparation stage, an observation readily acknowledged by DiClemente & Prochaska (1998); similarly, concern about confidence matters can also arise in the contemplation stage, as we discovered in experimental consultations with smokers (see Chapter 2, p. 20). Narrow stage-dose thinking, which restricts our attention in the contemplation stage only to matters of importance (pros and cons) could undermine the value of the stages of change model.

Linking *motivational* struggles to concerns about importance, whatever the person's stage of change, might also be ill advised. It implies that those concerned about confidence building do not experience motivational problems. Guided by this assumption, practitioners can be tempted simply to provide these patients with a few pieces of advice. The outcome is usually a motivational struggle and resistance from the patient. Motivational interviewing, a specialist method developed for preparing people for change, is not confined to matters of importance, but also embraces difficulties with confidence building. The term motivation itself, we have suggested (see Chapter 2, p. 23), should embrace both importance and confidence issues and be defined as equivalent to the more general concept of readiness to change.

Whither matching?

The above discussion has centered around this idea of matching using the stages of change model. Can this notion be rescued from the kind of narrow stage-dose thinking described above?

Researchers have looked at matching interventions to stages quite carefully, a good example being the Project MATCH study, i.e. will those who are less ready to change do better with a form of motivational interviewing; and, conversely, will those who are more ready do better with a cognitive–behavioral approach? The results of this kind of study have been mixed (see Rollnick 1998). An alternative pragmatic approach is to use generally tailored versus standardized interventions, in the hope of demonstrating that using the stages of change 'approach' is better than a more conventional approach to intervention. Reviews of this work can be found in Ashworth (1997) and DiClemente & Prochaska (1998). There is certainly something in this idea of matching according to readiness, but the findings could be stronger.

We have already suggested that an oversimplified notion of people's needs in different stages might account for these mixed results. Certainly, we would suggest that using the concepts of importance and confidence as matching criteria instead of, or in addition to, the concept of readiness, might be more constructive and avoid some of these oversimplifications.

Could it also be, however, that these studies of matching are too far removed from what actually goes on in the consulting room, and that the concept of matching is itself troublesome? As practitioners we would say, 'Yes!' Matching is not best achieved by giving a predefined dose of intervention to patients, but by responding to changing needs on an ongoing basis in the consultation. In this sense, we could view matching simply as a process of maintaining *congruence* in the consultation (Rollnick 1998). Sometimes a contemplator likes to talk about the importance of change; at other times about confidence. The same applies to people in the preparation stage. No wonder, then, that it has been difficult to locate matching effects in the studies by Heather et al (1996) and the Project MATCH team.

If these observations have some validity, the implications for trainers and practitioners are clear-cut: avoid oversimplified definitions of stages and interventions. It is similarly unwise to talk about a 'stage of change approach', as if this is a single method or intervention. In truth, we are talking about the delicate matter of how patients are spoken to, and about what specific changes they feel most ready to tackle. The best match is therefore not in some measurable characteristic of a patient, like readiness, or in some prepackaged intervention, but right inside the consulting room, with the practitioner attempting to maintain congruence with the patient.

Importance and confidence: some conceptual roots

In Chapter 2 we made a distinction between importance (the 'why' of change) and confidence (the 'how' of change) for understanding a person's expressed readiness to change. This emerged not just from thinking about consultations, but from a scrutiny of the literature, where we encountered a bewildering range of overlapping theories; for example, reasoned action, self-efficacy, health beliefs, decisional balance and subjective expected utility theory, all of which looked at the question of why and how people change their behavior. It soon became clear that there is no single model that adequately explains the sometimes baffling complexity of behavior change (Butler et al 1996). Neither is there one theory which is close to being uniformly endorsed by researchers and theorists. We decided, however, that in self-efficacy theory there was a useful framework which overlapped with many others.

Bandura (1977) developed a theory of behavior change based on two central concepts, efficacy and outcome expectations, but he then placed almost exclusive emphasis on the former during the next two decades. Efficacy expectations (or self-efficacy) refer to a person's confidence in his or her ability to master a particular behavior change in a variety of circumstances, hence our decision to use the term 'confidence'. This is not the same as a general concept like 'self-confidence'. Self-efficacy refers to a specific change, and to the person's sense of confidence about coping with specific circumstances. Outcome expectations, on the other hand, refer to judgments about whether the change in question will lead to valued outcomes, hence our decision to use the term 'importance'. In other words, someone is more likely to change a given behavior if he or she believes that, on balance, it will lead to good outcomes (outcome expectations) and that, across a range of situations, he or she will be able to master the skills needed to achieve that change (efficacy expectations).

References to the concept of outcome expectation abound in other models of behavior change. For example, reasoned action theory, the health belief model and the decisional balance model have used different terms to describe a similar terrain: how people make judgments about the importance or value of behavior change. It is with some relief that we have encountered a more recent model which embraces both the concept of self-efficacy and these outcome expectations of the value of change (see Schwartzer & Fuchs 1995, 1996).

Having made a distinction between the 'why' and 'how' of change, there is nothing like a good dose of clinical reality to completely blur the distinction between them. Sometimes they do seem quite distinct, for example, when the perceived importance of change is markedly low while confidence is high. This is illustrated by a heavy drinker who anticipates no difficulty in reducing consumption (high confidence), but who does not feel that such a change would be worthwhile (low perceived importance). At other times the two concepts interrelate, particularly when perceived importance is relatively high and confidence is low. Many smokers, for example, would very much like to quit but do not value the idea of change precisely because of the unpleasant perceived outcomes of coping with abstinence in difficult situations (i.e. low levels of perceived confidence). Moreover, as someone becomes increasingly ready to change, the 'why' and 'how' questions can collide, as reflected in the exasperation of someone who shrugs and says, 'No, I just can't do it, it's not worth it'. However, our clinical experience tells us that this does not render the distinction worthless.

Is behavior change always beneficial?

If a patient succeeds with change, is this always a good idea? Practitioners vary considerably in their views about this, because they, like their patients, differ in how much value they place on maintaining good health and preventing future illness.

For some people, given their unique circumstances, change might be counterproductive. Advising a terminally ill patient with lung cancer to quit smoking might be one rather extreme example. To take another, what would we say to one of the world's most famous classical guitarists who recently offered these reflections about his life? 'I probably eat, drink and smoke more than I should, but then I enjoy life immensely which probably evens things out … Nicotine slightly raises blood pressure, stimulating the red corpuscles under the finger nails, encouraging them to grow. On occasions when I have briefly stopped smoking, the tone of my playing has lost its bloom, because the nails are considerably weakened.' (*The Guardian*, 14 January 1997). The method in this book is based on the assumption that the patient is usually the best judge of whether behavior change will be beneficial. The observation of resistance, for example, provides a signal that we might be placing greater value on change than the patient does.

Sometimes, the decision to talk about behavior change with a patient is influenced by a policy to effect change in as many patients as possible. Two examples below suggest that sometimes this effort might not always be worthwhile, that patients are sometimes prematurely encouraged to consider change.

Pressure from the action-oriented clinic: the neglect of more important matters

Patients can rush into premature behavior change, aided by well-meaning practitioners and the setting in which they work. For example, in a cardiac rehabilitation setting, a perfectly compliant patient is defined as one who sets about health behavior change as soon as possible. This understandable and admirable reaction in patients can be therapeutic and lasting, but in other cases it is premature. Some might have other issues that should be addressed first, for example feelings of loss and fears about dying. The behavior change quite often overrides attention to these issues, and could be one explanation for relapse.

We recently heard an account of patients in a spinal injuries unit which illustrates this point very well, one which we believe is mirrored in other settings like cardiac rehabilitation clinics: two men had reacted in unison to the trauma of their terrible injuries. They set about exercising their arms and other muscles in an almost frenetic way. The comment from a psychologist was, *This is just the honeymoon phase, unfortunately. The next stage is depression, when they realize that they won't recover the function of their legs at all. Then they will start to resist the efforts of the physiotherapists. What they need is to talk about loss.* The staff were understandably not trained to deal with these subtle disparities between behavioral and emotional adaptation. Premature behavior change in some patients can be just as unproductive as the pervading helplessness which prevents efforts to change in others. In either case, skills in helping with adaptation to loss are just as relevant as skills in negotiating behavior change.

Probably more common is the example of a clinic in which the practitioners promote premature behavior change which is firmly resisted by many of the patients. Again, our hypothesis is that there is an underlying issue which is cast aside by the clinic as secondary to promoting behaviour change.

Marco suffers from what the doctors and nurses call asthma. He's been coming to the clinic for some years, and regularly hears talk about behavior change. For example, 'Remember not only to take your inhaler, but also the other medicine' [*a prophylactic steroid*]. Marco seldom takes this advice. The practitioners feel frustrated about his poor compliance and apparent irrationality.

Many patients like Marco have concerns about what they see as the dangers in taking a particular medicine like a steroid. This is not a particularly deep underlying issue, and one is left wondering whether the patient's concerns about taking medicine are dealt with through information exchange in a sufficiently thorough manner at the point of diagnosis. More serious, however, is the fact that Marco does not agree that he has asthma in the first place. He calls it his 'bad chest'. Lack of agreement about the meaning and implications of a diagnosis could account for quite a lot of poor compliance, something which came to light in a recent study of patients with asthma (Adams et al 1997). Time spent talking with Marco about exactly what the diagnosis means and how this fits into his everyday life might have prevented so much time and effort being wasted in repeated exhortations to take his medicine as prescribed. The focus by the clinic staff on behavior change (taking medicine) was clearly premature in Marco's case.

Pressure from the public health lobby

Practitioners face pressure to consider patient behavior change from many directions: from families, from patients themselves, from their own genuine concern for the person's health, and so on. One source of pressure is from the arena of public health which views health promotion in the consulting room as an excellent opportunity to change the behavior of large numbers of people, hence the rationale for many of the 'brief intervention' studies carried out in primary care over the last 20 years. In one of the first smoking studies in primary care, Russell et al (1979) asserted that, 'The results suggest that any GP who adopts this simple routine could expect about 25 long-term successes yearly. If all GPs in the UK participated the yield would exceed half a million ex-smokers a year' (p. 239). Studies among excessive drinkers followed soon after. In one of the largest and most carefully conducted, Wallace and colleagues (1988, p. 667) conclude, 'Our findings suggest that if all general practitioners were to participate actively in preventative intervention ... 250,000 men and 67,500 women [in the UK] would reduce their consumption to moderate levels'. Put simply, the message here is that practitioners should change their behavior (more screening and intervening) in order to change the behavior of their patients, *even if the large majority of recipients of brief intervention do not respond* (true for all of these brief intervention studies).

Is this utilitarian approach to health promotion as clear and as trouble-free as the literature suggests? Have practitioners complied with these exhortations? The intervention, usually a variant of advice-giving, is assumed to be simple and innocuous, and a conflict between the priorities of public health and the needs of individuals is simply not discussed in this literature (Rollnick et al 1997b). It is unfortunate that most of this effort proceeded without first asking practitioners and patients what they thought of it. The results of a few studies have trickled in with messages that are far from enthusiastic: practitioners talk about concerns about time, damaging the doctor–patient relationship and invading patient privacy (Wechsler et al 1983, Bruce & Burnett 1991, Coulter & Schofield 1991, Arborelius & Thakker 1995, Rollnick et al 1997b). Patients, for their part, apparently have reservations about being told what to do (Stott & Pill 1990). One study of smokers suggests that many feel overwhelmed by information and advice, resulting in feelings of guilt, irritation and the modification of help-seeking behavior in response to repeated advice about lifestyle change (Butler et al 1998). The problem is this: when the public health message enters the consulting room it does not *necessarily* coincide with the needs of the practitioner and the patient. To believe that talking about behavior change to patients is always a good idea is to risk entertaining an oversimplified view of what happens in the consulting room. There are times when, for very good reasons, behavior change is not on the agenda.

In deciding whether to raise the subject of behavior change, practitioners juggle with a host of questions. Do I have the time? Will I be successful? Is this the right time for the patient? What strategy should I use? Will there be conflict? In the face of this complexity, a practitioner's decision to leave behavior change to one side should not be viewed as a compliance problem, to be tackled with ever more incisive ways of 'getting the public health message across' to practitioners. Decontextualized health promotion interventions aimed at practitioners will meet with the same fate as decontextualized interventions delivered to patients: only a few will respond, for understandable reasons (Rollnick et al 1997b). Sometimes behavior change is viable and valued; at other times not.

It should be clear from this discussion that our vantage point is the consulting room and the well-being of the practitioner and patient. Our conclusion is that when health promotion is attempted, advice-giving, as conceived in the brief intervention literature, could lead to conflict because patients might feel pressurized in a situation in which the context of their behavior and concerns about it are not really tackled. It is our hope that the method outlined in this book will enable practitioners to tread the path between public health priorities and individual needs with greater sensitivity and efficacy.

Social versus psychological models of behavior change

The ideas in this book for guiding talk about behavior change are explicitly psychological, yet we know that unhealthy behavior is often maintained by social and environmental forces largely beyond the control of the practitioner, and to varying degrees, beyond the control of the individual. Our limited impact on a host of social forces like stress, disadvantage and family problems is a regular source of frustration. We are not social engineers, and we cannot enter people's homes to support them in efforts to change their behavior. We cannot, therefore, expect to be supremely successful with efforts in the consulting room. Faced with these humbling observations, it is often tempting for practitioners to leave the matter of healthy habits and lifestyles to the experts in public health. Unfortunately there is no escape. The effects of disadvantage, disability, stress and family problems permeate clinics and surgeries. Along with them come behavioral problems.

Where does this leave psychological models of behavior change? This is a complex matter. Generalization about the importance of social versus psychological models is difficult, because their relevance varies across individuals and circumstances. It is probably not helpful to create a false dichotomy. Our conclusion is that, despite the obvious impact of social forces, if someone is sitting in front of you, you are obliged to work with the psychological: the feelings and aspirations of the individual, and the interpersonal forces between you and the patient. This does not mean, however, that social matters are ignored. A patient carries into the consulting room an almost visible set of social circumstances. *The psychological expectations of this person are not separate from these broader contextual matters. They are often expressions of it.* For example, 'I cannot think about change at the moment. I can't even get the hot water cylinder repaired.' The concepts of readiness, importance and confidence are useful to the extent that they allow the practitioner to understand social context. Adopting a patient-centered consulting style involves heightened sensitivity to social and environmental pressures on individual patients. A useful theory of behavior change or method derived from it should allow one to enter the social world through the eyes of the individual.

Compliance, concordance and the role of authority

We have noted in a number of places that we reject the conceptual framework that surrounds the use of the term *compliance*, since it contains the mistaken assumption that behavior change (usually taking medication) will follow from the clear delivery of expert information to the relatively passive patient (see Butler et al 1996). The method described in this book is much more compatible with other frameworks like that based on concordance in which the patient's context is taken into account and he or she is encouraged to be an active decision-maker. The vehicle for doing this, we believe, is by maintaining *congruence* in the consultation with the patient's feelings and attitude to change. In more traditional terms, this will lead to better compliance rates. However, we do not propose this model just because it will lead to better results, but because we place high value on respect for patients' autonomy.

Care should be taken not to become complacent in the use of this concept of congruence. It can lead to an appeal to the moral high ground, in which adherents indulge in the coincidence between apparently effective methods and a value system which emphasizes patient autonomy. Dogmatism and oversimplification are usually not far away. One example is the notion that *any* appeal to or use of the practitioner's authority is a bad thing, incompatible with the overriding principle of ensuring patient freedom of decision making. Unfortunately, however, the shift from compliance to congruence, however well-meant this might be, can never free the practitioner from the role of authority which pervades the consultation. It is built into the fabric of healthcare. Indeed, one can argue that this authority is a potentially powerful force for healing, something many patients expect and want. Practitioners thus need to find a way of harnessing their authority in the best interests of the patients.

Matters of authority will invade the most delicate and humane efforts to maintain congruence and, vice versa, the most strident advice-giving to ensure compliance can be filled with sensitivity. There is no one way to achieve behavior change. What we have done in this book is try to provide guidelines for good practice in a field where, in truth, there is no escape from the issues of authority and autonomy.

Responsibility

A nurse strongly adheres to the principles of a patient-centered approach to behavior change. Giving patients choice, encouraging open discussion of the struggles and triumphs is what he enjoys when talking to patients. He does not believe that he should impose his desire for change on patients, but does feel that a jointly agreed plan of action should be pursued. His role is to provide useful information and support. Responsibility for deciding about change, in other words, should be shared. A patient with diabetes comes in for a routine check-up. She believes she has an illness, and that it is the responsibility of the nurses and doctors to provide all the help they can. The nurse raises the subject of lifestyle behavior change, and the patient immediately feels blamed. She thinks, but does not say, *'I see, so now it's my fault I have this illness'*. And the most well-meant effort from the nurse stumbles on the issue of responsibility. A resigned look comes over the patient and the nurse wonders where to go next.

Behavior change consultations often revolve around the issue of responsibility. Patients expect practitioners to provide treatment and solutions for health problems: after all, that is what they are trained to do. However, if some of the solutions to a problem (e.g. heart disease) lie in health behavior change, how can a practitioner be responsible for that? If this is the main stage on which talk about behavior change is played out, there are numerous other smaller happenings which also raise the subject of responsibility: who should decide how to structure the consultation, what topic to talk about, what information to exchange, what medicines to take and what the patient should actually do about behavior change.

Our assumption in this book has been that the practitioner should provide structure to the consultation; and information, keeping a firm eye on the reactions and aspirations of the patient. We have also assumed that responsibility for *decision making in the consultation* should not reside with the practitioner, but should be a joint effort, with emphasis being placed on the patient's freedom of choice about behavior change. However, even if we are guided by this kind of patient-centered framework, conflict over responsibility will not be avoided. Patients will not necessarily hold consistent and uniform views about the wide range of questions noted above.

The goal of a patient-centered method and the use of concepts like resistance is to encourage sensitivity to areas of potential disagreement. It can be helpful always to bear in mind two questions: *What does this patient feel responsible for?* and *What does he or she feel is my responsibility?* Using this approach does not mean handing over responsibility for all matters to the patient. It means working out who takes responsibility for what decision inside and outside the consulting room.

'I want this and you want that': more complex consultations

It is one thing to deal with the complexity of a patient's decision making, but it becomes more difficult when the practitioner also feels pressure from the patient to make decisions and to change his or her own behavior.

All the concepts and methods we have described thus far have a notably one-sided focus on the patient's feelings and behavior. How, then, do we understand and deal with those frequently occurring situations where the need for change is exerted from both directions? (The statements below reflect not what practitioner and patient actually say to each other, but what they might feel about the consultation.

Sore throat

Patient: *I want an antibiotic.*

Practitioner: *I want you to learn to cope with this kind of condition on your own.*

Minor ailment

Patient: *I want a 'sick note'* [so I can stay off work].

Practitioner: *Take this treatment and you should be better very soon.*

Chronic pain

Patient: *I want you to help me with pain relief (and a complete cure for my pain).*

Practitioner: *I want you to do these exercises (and accept that you have a lifelong, chronic condition).*

Chronic fatigue

Patient: *I want a diagnosis and treatment.*

Practitioner: *I would like you to take charge and do a number of things to help yourself to get better.*

Addiction

Patient: *I need help for 'my nerves'* [a tranquilizer] *and new housing* [a letter from you to the Housing Department].

Practitioner: *You really must stop drinking.*

Probation office

Client: *I need you to help me avoid a prison sentence.*

Practitioner: *If you stopped using drugs you would have better control over your life.*

In Chapter 6 we have described how one might deal with potentially conflict-ridden encounters of this kind (see pp. 156–167). However, we are aware of the one-sided nature of our suggested approach. In truth, concepts like resistance, readiness, importance and confidence can be applied to both parties. In each of the consultations cited above, one can imagine at least two readiness continua, with practitioner and patient potentially at opposite ends of each of them. Further development work will be needed to construct a framework which takes into account the subtle tensions created by pressure for change moving in both directions. Even the concept of rapport might need to be refined: one can imagine rapport being quite good when one topic is discussed, but almost absent when talk turns to another. Staying on a 'good wavelength' with a patient will require awareness of strong feelings on both sides and considerable negotiating skill.

Our experience of studying one of these types of consultation, the 'sore throat' encounter, reveals that conflict does not necessarily emerge, despite strong feelings on both sides. Rather, practitioner and patient seem to steer a path through them in which conflict is avoided and both parties are respectful to one another (Butler et al, 1998). Yet practitioners describe this as the most uncomfortable prescribing decision they are faced with (Bradley 1992). Contextual forces on both sides can swing the decision to prescribe either way: for example, if the doctor is tired and short of time, and the patient is perceived as under stress more generally, prescribing is probably a more likely outcome.

One doctor who we interviewed said, 'I arrived here [in this clinic] and despite numerous attempts to address the situation, we seem to have failed … we've all thrown in the towel … Most of them [the patients] will not take no for an answer, at the end of the day you [could] spend 15 minutes trying to educate them, when you know they will go out disillusioned, come back the next day and see someone else, making you feel 5 minutes would be better spent just giving them a prescription and getting rid of them. It's an awful thing to say, but it's true. … The worst area of clinical practice in terms of good clinical medicine is the prescribing of antibiotics for URTI (coughs, colds and sore throats)' (Butler et al 1998). This doctor was a high prescriber. Another, working in very similar circumstances, found a different solution: she constructed an algorithm on her computer, into which the patient's symptoms were entered. When the computer came back with the answer 'no need for antibiotics', she would turn to the patient, shrug her shoulders, and say, 'The computer, which takes into account your symptoms and the latest evidence, says I should not prescribe'. The patients were apparently much more likely to accept this recommendation.

In some of the consultations listed above, for example, chronic fatigue and chronic pain, patients usually make their expectations quite clear, thus presenting the practitioner with the possibility of open conflict. In contrast, in the sore throat consultations, we found that, out of a total of 37 practitioners and patients we interviewed, only one patient said that she had expressed the desire for antibiotics, and only one doctor said that he routinely asked patients what they wanted.

This 'two-way' talk about behavior change is therefore not a simple matter. We believe, however, that there should be room for improving the way in which these consultations are dealt with to the greater satisfaction of both parties.

CALLS FROM THE CONSULTING ROOM

What about relapse?

This topic has not been covered in this book, either in theory or practice. Where does this leave the practitioner facing a patient who has relapsed, a very common experience?

We are not convinced that it is essential to construct a different theoretical framework for understanding relapse, in addition to using the concepts of readiness, importance and confidence. Are we not talking about someone who, having relapsed, has merely become ready to do something else which we call relapse, i.e. a return to drinking, smoking, and so on? So too, if such a person is taking stock of the situation with a practitioner, he or she is facing a decision where surely the same three forces are at work. They are just in a different position in the cycle of change.

It might be useful to supplement this framework with some of the concepts developed in the specialist addictions field for understanding relapse. For example, the precipitants of relapse (mood states, social situations, etc.) have been extensively studied, and this might help patients understand why and how their behavior changed. We would, however, caution against the construction of a specialist arm of the behavior change field, for fear that this could undermine the value of focusing on the common processes across behavior change discussions. It could lead, for example, to the kind of stage-dose thinking which implies that those who relapse need a different form of intervention.

From a practical viewpoint, our preference would be for the use of a few relapse-specific strategies which fall within the same overall framework, but which allow the practitioner to talk about the topic in a constructive way. Here, there is considerable scope for development work. For example, is it a good idea to focus on the failures of the past? How can one examine relapse precipitants in a brief encounter, without reinforcing helplessness? Policing the past is a fairly commonly used strategy in clinics for the treatment of chronic conditions like diabetes. Under what circumstances is it better to start afresh, and ask the person, 'Where do we go from here?' (Stott et al 1995).

Some patients like to be told what to do

All practitioners can tell stories about patients who are passive and expectant of expert opinion. Indeed, in many cultures this kind of passivity is required of the person consulting a healer, witchdoctor or health practitioner. Surely the more negotiation-based method described here is inappropriate for some people, who perhaps might not want to take responsibility for sharing decision making? Unfortunately, we have not found a brief method for assessing at the outset of a discussion whether or not patients like to be told what to do when it comes to behavior change. If we had, we would be in a much better position to understand how many people feel this way, in what circumstances and how best to respond to them.

Care should be taken not to polarize the difference between advice-giving and a more negotiation-based approach to behavior change. This issue was discussed in Chapter 2. We have all given advice and told people what they should do without undermining their autonomy. Often this depends on how you say things. Similarly, we have also felt free to say what we think patients should do while guided by a more negotiation-based framework. We simply make sure that we emphasize their freedom to make a decision for themselves. In truth, if you have sufficiently good rapport with patients, you can usually tell them what you think they should do without any harm being done. Our concern about advice-giving is that it should not be the *guiding framework* for behaviour change consultations, because too many patients do not respond well. If you feel that a particular patient wants to be told what to do, try it and look out for resistance. If you are not sure, ask the patient.

Some patients will never change

Why should I be so optimistic about change? Some of my patients will never be able to. (*Dietician, aged 42*)

This kind of question echoes through our minds in every clinic, and the answer, we believe, is in the rejection of dogmatism. The problem is this: we are often quick to pass judgment, and we are often wrong. For example, our team of three counsellors once made a rating of each of 142 male heavy drinkers, at the receiving end of a hospital-based health promotion effort, i.e. 0 = very unlikely to change, 5 = very likely to change. Follow-up at 6 months revealed no relationship between our judgments and outcome. Some of the 'hopeless cases' did very well.

Yet we all know cases where our intuitions are borne out by seeing the same person, time after time, never changing. For example, a 55-year-old obese woman has been suffering, like her father before her, with the complications of diabetes. She routinely attends the clinic, submits herself to all the measurements, yet develops a blank look whenever one talks about dietary change. She struggles with a stressful and economically deprived lifestyle and, like her father before her, does not appear to believe that it is possible or worthwhile to slow the progress of the disease. The family value system is like a brick wall, and one shudders at the thought of what medical crisis might befall her.

It is one thing to feel resigned about a particular patient, but care should be taken in generalizing too much about peoples' chances, lest we develop hardened attitudes which are not in the interests of good practice. The method described in this book is not a panacea, imbued with healing powers to resolve problems like those described in the example above. It is, however, a method which calls for flexibility and the avoidance of dogmatism.

They know all the facts, but they never listen, they never change

This is probably the most frequently vented frustration in the treatment of chronic diseases like asthma, heart disease and diabetes. Patients are not short of information, in fact they often hear the same story about 'looking after yourself' in every clinic, yet they make very little progress in altering lifestyle habits.

There is obviously no single explanation or single answer to this problem. We have been very impressed by the way in which practitioners sometimes take a deep breath and decide to have an open discussion about the matter. The strategies in this book are merely aids to this activity (e.g. agenda setting, exploring importance). Perhaps the most surprising issue uncovered by these practitioners is that the patient is struggling not with behavior change, but with the meaning of the chronic disease itself. The case of Marco described above (p. 194) is a good example of this. Practitioners were prematurely talking about behavior change when Marco did not see 'the disease' in the same way as them. Along similar lines, we recently came across a 55-year-old man who had been diagnosed with insulin-dependent diabetes at the age of 11 years (see p. 24). Until very recently, he had been ignoring his disease, trying to live life despite it – as he put it, 'messing around with my insulin levels'. On his own admission, he behaved like an irritable and obnoxious person when he went to his routine clinic. He hated the way 'they' were obsessed by insulin levels. Then recently, a nurse and doctor decided that his physical condition was so serious that they had to take a different approach, give him more time, and allow him to talk about whatever he wanted to. They said that he had been in a state of 'denial' for over 40 years, not able to see the connection between his condition and his health problems. He said that they had given him 'help, not lectures', and that they had taken him 'into the real world', where he felt much more in control of what he wanted from life. The lesson seems clear enough: if patients repeatedly fail to 'listen' and to change, it might be worthwhile listening to them, without prejudice, to give them a chance to say what truly underlies their apparent disengagement from the agenda of the practitioner.

A little bit of knowledge can be dangerous

I attended a workshop and you encouraged me to examine why my patients are unsure about change. I did this, unpacked a lot of personal issues, then I got stuck and did not know how to end the brief consultation effectively. Don't you think that's dangerous? (*Community nurse, aged 27*)

At least three issues emerge from this comment, each worthy of being taken seriously. These are: first, that we might endanger patients; second, that practitioners might be harmed by feeling out of their depth, and third, that a one-off training experience can leave practitioners feeling inadequately supported.

First, one can imagine a scenario in which concern about harming patients is legitimate. A practitioner with poor communication skills uses a behavior change strategy like a dose of intervention with a poor sense of timing and judgment, and leaves the patient feeling upset. We have taken care to emphasize the spirit of this method (Chapter 2), which is based upon listening carefully and working with the readiness to change of the patient. As such, used with a modicum of skill, it can do patients no harm. The nurse described above is not likely to do any harm because he is asking questions of his own consulting behavior and watching the reaction of his patients. The chances are that his judgment will improve with time, experience and support.

The second issue, practitioners feeling out of their depth, is a serious challenge which faces trainers and supervisors. Use of this method can and does leave practitioners feeling out of their depth at times. We know a nurse who said that it took about a year before she felt comfortable with an adjustment to her consulting style and felt at home with a more flexible approach to behavior change. During this period she struggled. Fortunately, one of us had the opportunity to talk to her about her experiences, which were as much positive as negative. The main difficulty was how to handle a situation in which both parties realized that there was no way out of an impasse: it simply was not the right time to consider change. This colleague's resolution of this problem involved feeling free to summarize the situation for the patient, and to offer reassurance that change takes time, that it is better to think things over before rushing into a decision. The battle was with her own sense of impotence to solve patients' problems for them. Our hunch is that feeling out of one's depth is a call for more supervision and training, not for a return to simple advice-giving.

The third problem, providing inadequate, one-off training, is a pervasive one, particularly in a relatively new field which has not been integrated into the basic training of practitioners in a widespread manner. However, the solution, we believe, is not to stop conducting one-off training workshops, but to do this in such a way that practitioners' concerns about skill levels are responded to with openness, reassurance, and some level-headed guidance about the sometimes tricky road ahead. Adherence to the guidelines presented in Chapter 7 should ensure that the limitations of one-off training are minimized. The impetus for writing this book came from a desire to prompt curriculum designers to place the subjects of behavior change and information exchange close to the top of the list in the basic training of practitioners. Until that happens, the concern of the nurse quoted above will be a legitimate one.

Why so much talk about behavior? What about feelings?

The focus on behavior in this book might appear to have a narrow and somewhat arbitrary quality to it. How can one separate behavior from attitudes and feelings? Why develop strategies specifically for dealing with behavior in the absence of accompanying guidelines for dealing with these other domains? One answer to this is that one has to make a start somewhere. Practitioners spend a lot of time on the specific topic of behavior change, and we believe that the quality of this activity could be much improved. However, *to view the tasks and strategies in this book as narrowly focused on behavior would be to misunderstand their function*. We have described a number of concepts, principles and strategies that help a practitioner to explore and acknowledge the way a patient is feeling and thinking. The patient-centered method is a critical foundation for ensuring that one does not stray into an oversimplified discussion of health behavior, removed from the personal context in which it occurs. Other concepts and strategies serve the same function: the observation of resistance, for example, is often a signal that the patient would prefer to talk about another issue; asking a patient about the importance of change sometimes directly leads to the exploration of a more fundamental personal matter. The agenda-setting task was deliberately designed to encourage the patient to talk about other concerns beyond behavior change.

Habits and addictions

A long-term heavy user of Valium will probably find it more difficult to change behavior than a young heavy drinker who is not dependent on alcohol. One of the differences between these two cases is in the degree of physical dependence on the substance. Remove the substance and the Valium user will experience withdrawal symptoms. Some people report severe symptoms which cripple their attempts to change and leave them feeling demoralized and trapped. Others, also apparently with a severe addiction, appear to find the transition from use to abstinence more straightforward. In the literature, debate about the meaning and ramifications of addiction has been smoldering for many years, particularly in the alcohol field (see Heather & Robertson 1989). This is not merely an academic debate, but one which has serious practical consequences.

Clearly, another inescapable difference between the long-term Valium user and the young heavy drinker is in their degree of attachment to the substance, independent of any physical components of addiction. Here we begin to move out of the realms of substance use. Do something for long enough, anything, and it can become a habit that is difficult to break. Sometimes the habit pervades many aspects of the person's daily life (e.g. gambling, drinking coffee, eating chocolate), and sometimes it is more circumscribed (e.g. brushing teeth). Obviously, *the consequences* vary across individuals and behaviors. As negative consequences emerge, if they do, the person can be become embroiled in conflict about whether to change or not.

In general, addiction can be viewed too narrowly as a matter of physical dependence, without sufficient emphasis being placed on habit strength and the patient's beliefs and moods. One of the consequences of this view, it could be argued, has been the emergence of specialists trained to help people through withdrawal and readjustment. This can be a double-edged sword. While intensive help is clearly extremely valuable for some people, particularly for those without active support in the community, it can reinforce the idea that a practitioner in a general healthcare setting is in no position to deal with such matters. We question this assumption. There will never be enough specialists to deal with the number of addictive problems that appear in primary and other general healthcare settings, something which policy makers have begun to take note of. Sufferers, for their part, might not necessarily want the perceived stigma and inconvenience of specialist referral. Most important, however, is our belief that practitioners can make a great deal of progress within the limited time available to them. We have found it possible to use the methods in this book with patients suffering from severe addiction problems.

Most of these patients actually change their behavior quite naturally, without help from anyone. The method described in this book can be used as a *starting point* with any kind of problem, be it someone seriously dependent on Valium, a long-term heavy smoker, a severe problem drinker or someone suffering from obesity. Whether this relatively brief input is sufficient is another matter, something for the patient and practitioner to decide about. Establishing rapport, often in the face of considerable guilt and remorse, can be a powerful first step. Helping a patient express how he or she really feels about the issue (i.e. by assessing importance and confidence) can sometimes precipitate spontaneous change. For their part, practitioners need to hang on to the most important observation to emerge from the stages of change model: that action is not the only measure of success in a consultation. In fact, for the majority this is inappropriate, because they are not ready for this, let alone for accepting the idea of specialist referral. Helping someone think about change is a critical process, well within the capability of the general healthcare practitioner. Addictive problems should not be mystified as being too complex. Whatever the degree of physical dependence, the challenges for the practitioner remain the same: establish rapport and have a constructive discussion about change.

METHODS AND THEIR EFFECTIVENESS

Motivational interviewing: how broad is the horizon?

Motivational interviewing is a specialist method developed in the addictions field for helping people with severe behavior change difficulties (Miller & Rollnick 1991, Rollnick & Miller 1995). Some parts of this book have been directly influenced by motivational interviewing, for example in the discussion of resistance, while others have emerged from general healthcare settings rather than the addiction field, for example strategies for agenda setting and the assessing of importance and confidence. In a very broad sense, however, all of the material in this book follows the main goal of motivational interviewing: patients should be encouraged to produce arguments for change, and ways of achieving it, rather than have these presented to them by the practitioner.

Why then, have we not simply called this method and book something like 'medical motivational interviewing' or 'brief motivational interviewing'? The problem is this: motivational interviewing is a *counseling style* which relies heavily on the use of reflective listening skills by specialists who are given time to learn these skills, and who often have hours rather than minutes to spend with their clients. They use motivational interviewing to explore sometimes deeply personal conflicts.

The average healthcare practitioner is in a quite different situation: much less time to acquire listening skills, a wide range of other responsibilities besides behavior change, and much less time with patients. Our emphasis has been upon readily teachable brief strategies which encourage practitioners to use listening skills. We do not believe, however, that it is realistic to expect them to use techniques like reflective listening to a uniformly high standard. Moreover, some of the elements of motivational interviewing are clearly beyond the scope of brief healthcare consultations. The principle of deploying discrepancy provides one example. Here the counselor helps the client to see the way in which his or her deeper values are at odds with some of the personally destructive consequences of a behavior problem like dependence on gambling or alcohol. A strategy based on this principle requires time and considerable care to avoid running into ethical difficulties. We would not teach this to healthcare practitioners, or encourage them to use it.

To call methods like those we have described 'medical motivational interviewing' could result in the premature use of strategies by practitioners who do not have recourse to adequate training and support. It would also serve to dilute what is a specialist counseling style.

Motivational interviewing has served as the inspiration for developments in a wide range of more specialist activities, from the treatment of sexual abusers (Mann & Rollnick 1996) to topics like eating disorders (Schmidt & Treasure 1997), compliance with psychiatric medication (Kemp et al 1996) and emergency room interventions (D'Onofrio et al 1996, Bernstein et al 1997). We hope that it continues to inspire developments in more general healthcare settings. A brief review of the evidence about the effectiveness of motivational interviewing can be found below (see p. 210).

Addiction counseling and its horizons

Are the strategies in this book of any use to specialists like addiction counselors? They might be, because many counseling sessions in the addictions field are brief, one-off affairs. How to make the most of the first contact is thus a critical consulting skill. Moreover, some of the strategies in this book, like *agenda setting* (Chapter 3, p. 46), might be of value in specialist settings where there is always a danger that the counselor might prematurely focus on his or her area of expertise, at the expense of keeping the focus broad to begin with. Finally, there is the question of skill acquisition in training. Our experience has been that teaching concrete strategies to specialist counselors (see Bell & Rollnick 1996), some of them described in this book, has some clear benefits: they go back to the workplace with clear guidelines for good practice.

Other methods

The strategies in this book could be greatly enhanced by integration with other methods which we have not had the opportunity to examine and pilot in healthcare settings. The world of counseling and therapy is undergoing a transformation in which adherence to strict schools of therapy is breaking down. Something called a brief therapy movement has also emerged (see de Shazer et al 1986, Barkham 1989, Iveson & Ratner 1990, Pinsoff 1994). These new approaches to brief consultations are not necessarily tied to a particular theory or model, but instead work on the assumption that brief counseling should start with the expectations of the client. A good example is the work on brief therapeutic consultations described by Street & Downey (1996). Here, one encounters a description of different patterns of help seeking by clients which could be of considerable benefit in the general healthcare consultation setting: intervention varies depending on whether the person is an advice seeker, opinion seeker, action expector or theory seeker. The work on brief therapy, much of which was developed while working with families, could be usefully integrated into the more narrowly defined brief we gave ourselves in this book: to focus on behavior change in the individual.

Closer to home, we have neglected to properly examine and develop the work of other colleagues in healthcare settings who have developed methods clearly relevant to behavior change. For example, Botelho (1992) and Keller and White (1997) have outlined useful models of negotiation for behavior change consultations.

Where is the evidence?

This question should rightly be asked of the strategies we have described. Care will need to be taken, however, in avoiding oversimplified answers.

There is no shortage of research on the theoretical question of how best to understand and predict behavior (see, for example, Ogden 1996). On the other hand, methods designed to encourage behavior change have not received the attention they deserve, given the importance of this for the prognosis of so many diseases. As we noted in the Preface (p. vii), we believe this is a result of insufficient attention being paid to developing behavior change methods in the first place.

Advice-giving

Most of the evidence that is available about health behavior change is confined to evaluations of brief advice-giving (see, for example, Ashenden et al 1997). Our conclusion is that research support does exist for health promotion work of this kind, but that the effect sizes are small, and there is not a lot of evidence that healthcare practitioners apply the findings of behavior change research on a widespread basis. The starting point for writing this book was that a generic method, which was not confined to a specific behavior, would be more attractive to practitioners because it would be applicable across different kinds of consultation and behavior change problems. It might also prove to be more effective if sufficient attention is given to enhancing the communication skills necessary to use it to a sufficiently high standard (Rollnick et al 1997b).

Motivational interviewing

Evaluation of the strategies described in this book should not be confused with evidence for the support of motivational interviewing, for the reasons noted previously on pages 207–208. Support for motivational interviewing has emerged in a number of settings. For example, a large number of studies have been carried out among problem drinkers (e.g. Miller et al 1988, 1993, Bien et al 1993, Brown & Miller 1993, Allsop et al 1997, Project MATCH Research Group 1997), while others have focused on drug users (Saunders et al 1995) and heavy drinkers (Heather et al 1996). Any review of this field will run into the problem of defining motivational interviewing, because adaptation in different settings (e.g. Kuchipudi et al 1988, Senft et al, 1995) can result in a dilution of the essence of the method (see Rollnick & Miller 1995). Reviewers will also vary in the conclusions they reach about effectiveness. Our impression is that there is evidence for effectiveness in some studies and some settings, but that our understanding of exactly why motivational interviewing seems to work, and how to improve it, still needs a great deal of attention.

The stages of change model

There is a danger that this model is viewed as equivalent to a single method of intervention, an assumption made by numerous practitioners and researchers who we have met. The problem is that no such intervention exists. Rather, Prochaska & DiClemente have deliberately constructed a transtheroetical *model* which is designed to embrace and explain the workings of a wide range of therapeutic interventions. Practitioners using the stages of change model as a guiding framework inevitably use a variety of interventions. Research on this model will be obliged to conduct more refined studies which look at the question of what kind of intervention is best suited to different stages of change. The strategies we have described have been strongly influenced by the stages of change model and the writing of Prochaska & DiClemente, but their effectiveness or otherwise should not be construed as providing direct evidence in support of the model.

The toolbox in this book

Researchers will not be able to easily ask the question 'does *it* work?' because this book does not contain one method, but a toolbox of strategies. The evidence collected thus far, gathered in three controlled trials, is summarized below:

- A menu of strategies has been evaluated among heavy drinkers in a health promotion study in a general hospital setting. Nurses receiving brief training used a menu of strategies which included *A Typical Day* (p. 112), *pros and cons* (p. 81), *exploring concerns* (p. 87), *information exchange* (p. 16) and a decision-making strategy similar to *Brainstorming solutions* (p. 97). The method, described fully elsewhere (Rollnick & Bell 1991, Rollnick et al 1992), was found to be more effective than receiving no brief counseling. There was also an indication in the findings that this toolbox was more effective than a skills-based approach *among patients who were less ready to change*. Among those who were ready to change, it did not seem to matter whether they received this method or the more skills-based approach (Heather et al 1996). This study was bedeviled by small cell sizes and the result should be regarded as provisional.
- *Agenda setting* (p. 46) was developed and evaluated among patients with chronic non-insulin dependent diabetes in primary care (Stott et al 1995, 1996). A randomized controlled trial was unable to demonstrate that an intervention based on this strategy was more effective than standard care (Pill et al 1998). These results emerged in contrast to the enthusiasm we encountered among some practitioners. Our conclusion is that this strategy has considerable potential, but much more time needs to be given to training practitioners before its value can be properly assessed. In the above trial, this amounted to an initial training of less than 1 hour. When practitioners used it they came face to face with the issue of handing responsibility for change over to the patient

(Pill & Rees in press), a sometimes radical shift in consulting style which is unlikely to be achieved in a short training period.

• *Assessing importance and confidence* and the associated scaling questions formed the basis of a smoking intervention toolbox which was taught in a brief training time to general practitioners in primary care (see Chapter 3, p. 60 for further details). Practitioners responded well to this method (Rollnick et al 1997). The modest but statistically significant results (Butler et al in press) suggest that if more time had been spent ensuring competence in training, the findings would have been stronger.

These findings suggest that more careful attention to practitioner competence levels should improve the effectiveness of strategies within this toolbox.

Guidelines for research

The most telling lesson we have learned from conducting the above studies is to avoid the view of behavior change methods as one would a tablet of medicine. It led to a desire to launch a controlled trial as soon as possible, on the assumption that there would be a uniformly high standard of delivery of the intervention.

Failure to pilot adequately can result in the rigorous evaluation of an ill-defined intervention carried out by practitioners who do not have the skill and commitment to make a significant difference to the lives of their patients. For example, helping practitioners to adjust and refine their consulting style is as big a challenge as helping patients change their lifestyle behaviors. A controlled trial in surgery would not go ahead if there was not a satisfactory level of competence in the surgeons taking part. The same standard should apply in this field. Evaluation of a toolbox of behavior change strategies should therefore ensure that:

• The study should be conducted in *phases*.
• The toolbox or method of intervention should be sensitive to the setting and properly piloted, paying attention to the reactions of both practitioners and patients. The strategies chosen should be adapted and refined, and then outlined in writing.
• The selection of practitioners needs careful thought. It might be advisable to use more committed practitioners to begin with, even if this is a biased sample, on the grounds that if the method is used effectively by this group, it can then be examined under harsher conditions among less committed practitioners.
• The method for training practitioners should be piloted. The length of training should be adequate, and training itself should include practice. Evidence of attainment of adequate competence levels should be collected.
• Evaluation in practice among patients should be divided into two

stages, the first involving examination of efficacy (*Is the method effective?*), the second looking at broader issues like, *Can the method be used in a sustained and cost-effective manner in everyday practice?*

- Qualitative data should be collected throughout this process, on the reactions of practitioners and patients to the method being used.

Health behavior change groups

Some practitioners will be interested in the use of groups in healthcare settings which focus on behavior change, based on the methods described in this book. Supporting evidence is lacking and our experience of this has been limited, but sufficient to realize that this is a field rich in promise. Our inclination is not to divide people up into groups depending on their readiness to change. This can be useful, and we have encountered services offering groups for precontemplators, contemplators, and so on. The problem here, not surprisingly, is that people jump in and out of stages quite easily.

To run a group which focuses on a particular problem or behavior (e.g. diabetes, panic, alcohol) offers rich potential for promoting behavior change, as well as some serious traps which undermine autonomy and decision-making. The opportunities for observing the success of others and gaining their support are well-known and powerful forces in the self-help process.

Some of our strategies, like information exchange, could be useful because they would encourage participants to respond personally to information presented in a neutral and non-threatening way. So, too, we have encountered group assessments of readiness (on a continuum) which generate useful discussion. Participants could also use the importance and confidence dimensions in the same way. Having said this, we imagine that such a group requires considerable skill to run, with the facilitator striking a balance between providing information and structure on the one hand, and managing the variety of individual responses on the other. For example, what should one do when a patient articulates all the reasons why change feels impossible? How does one avoid being confrontational or dismissive in response to this? Practitioners who run such groups would need to be properly trained and supported and to follow guidelines for good practice which have emerged from careful pilot work.

Behavior change discussion in other settings and in everyday life

It is tempting to observe the parallels between behavior change discussions in the consulting room and in everyday life. Between these two lie a host of other contexts in which this topic is also relevant: schools, business settings, occupational health departments, gymnasiums, public health education institutes, political settings, and so on. People talk about behavior change, and often there is one or more people who would like to encourage change in others.

There is no reason in principle why the concepts and methods we describe should not be explored in these settings. Slavish application, however, is bound to run into trouble. In some settings, people are forced to change their behavior, for example, when obliged to adopt new work practices. This raises new issues which have not been tackled in sufficient detail in this book. In other settings, the dynamics might be quite different, where there is little or no obligation at all to change behavior, for example, when a parent approaches an 18-year-old about behavior change.

Behavior change discussions are likely to vary on other dimensions. For example, when one moves away from the relatively secure encounter with the individual, and embraces groups of people who vary in their readiness to change, one encounters fresh challenges, as one of us did when talking with 40 disaffected machine operators in a large company. The ideas and strategies in this book were useful to the extent that one could retain attachment to the following principle of behavior change: people are more likely to change their behavior if they are given time to explore the why and how of change for themselves, and not have this explained to them by an authority figure. So, too, a premature focus on action talk, when the majority are less ready to change, will generate resistance.

CONCLUSION

For all sorts of reasons, practitioners end up talking about behavior change. Support from textbooks and training curricula has been minimal, largely because attention has focused on specific pathologies (diabetes, heart disease) or behaviors (smoking, diet) at the expense of the pervasive common elements across consultations. The activity at the very heart of the matter is all too often guided by a crude combination of common sense, direct persuasion, simple advice and fearful information. No wonder then that wise practitioners develop artful strategies for themselves to avoid the subject of behavior change.

The strategies we describe in this book are not always a quick and easy route through this passage. The magic bullet does not exist. Yet we have found ourselves working well with patients, when the challenge of behavior change is well met by the use of strategies which guide purposeful conversation about change. These strategies should remain as just guidelines, and should never be allowed to dictate talk about change.

REFERENCES

Adams S, Pill R, Jones A 1997 Medication, chronic illness and identity; the perspective of people with asthma. Social Science and Medicine 45:189–201

Allsop S, Saunders B, Phillips M, Carr A 1997 A trial of relapse prevention with severely dependent male problem drinkers. Addiction 92:61–74

Annis H, Schober R, Kelly E 1996 Matching addiction outpatient counseling to client readiness for change: the role of structured relapse prevention counseling. Experimental and Clinical Psychopharmacology 4:37–45

Arborelius E, Thakker K D 1995 Why is it so difficult for general practitioners to discuss alcohol with their patients. Family Practice 12:419–422

Ashenden R, Silagy C, Weller D 1997 A systematic review of the effectiveness of promoting lifestyle change in general practice. Family Practice 14:160–176

Ashworth P 1997 Breakthrough or bandwagon? Are interventions tailored to stage of change more effective than non-staged interventions? Health Education Journal 56:166–174

Bandura A 1977 Towards a unifying theory of behavior change. Psychological Review 84:191–215

Bandura A 1995 Moving into forward gear in health promotion and disease prevention. Keynote address presented at the annual meeting of the Society of Behavioral Medicine 23 March 1995, San Diego

Barkham M 1989 Exploratory therapy in 2+1 sessions: 1. Rationale for a brief psychotherapy model. British Journal of Psychotherapy 6:81–88

Bell A, Rollnick S 1995 Motivational interviewing in practice: a structured approach. In: Rotgers F (ed) Treating substance abuse: theory and technique. Guilford Press, New York

Bernstein E, Bernstein J, Levenson S 1997 Project Assert: an ed-based intervention to increase access to primary care preventive services and the substance abuse treatment system. Annals of Emergency Medicine 30:181–189

Bien T, Miller W, Boroughs J 1993 Motivational interviewing with alcohol outpatients. Behavioural & Cognitive Psychotherapy 21:347–356

Botelho R 1992 A negotiation model for the doctor–patient relationship. Family Practice 9:210–218

Bradley C P 1992 Uncomfortable prescribing decisions: a critical incident study. British Medical Journal 304:294–296

Brown J, Miller W 1993 Impact of motivational interviewing on participation in residential alcoholism treatment. Psychology of Addictive Behaviours 7:211–218

Bruce N, Burnett S 1991 Prevention of lifestyle-related disease: general practitioners' views about their role, effectiveness and resources. Family Practice 8:373–377

Butler C C, Pill R, Stott N C H 1998 A qualitative study of patients' perceptions of doctors' advice to quit smoking: implications for opportunistic health promotion. British Medical Journal 316:1878–1881

Butler C C, Rollnick S, Stott N C H 1996 The practitioner, the patient and resistance to change: recent ideas on compliance. Canadian Medical Association Journal 154:1357–1362

Butler C C, Rollnick S, Cohen D, Russell I, Bachmann M, Stott N (in press) Motivational consulting versus brief advice for smokers in general practice: a randomised trial. British Journal of General Practice

Butler C C, Rollnick S, Pill R, Maggs-Rapport F, Stott N 1998 Understanding the culture of prescribing: a qualitative study of general practitioners' and patients' perceptions of antibiotics for sore throats. British Medical Journal 317:637–642

Coulter A, Schofield T 1991 Prevention in general practice: the views of doctors in the Oxford region. British Journal of General Practice 41:140–143

Davies P 1979 Motivation, responsibility and sickness in the psychiatric treatment of alcoholism. British Journal of Psychiatry 134:449–458

Davies P 1981 Expectations and therapeutic practices in outpatient clinics for alcohol problems. British Journal of Addiction 76:159–173

D'Onofrio G, Bernstein E, Rollnick S 1996 Motivating patients for change: a brief strategy for negotiation. In: Bernstein E, Bernstein J (eds) Case studies in emergency medicine and the health of the public. Jones & Bartlett, Massachusetts

de Shazer S, Berg I, Lipchick E, Nunnally E, Molnar A, Gingerich W, Weiner-Davies M 1986 Brief therapy: a focused solution development. Family Process 25:207–222

DiClemente C C 1991 Motivational interviewing and the stages of change. In: Miller W R, Rollnick S (eds) Motivational interviewing. Guilford Press, New York

DiClemente C C, Prochaska J 1998 Toward a comprehansive, transtheoretical model of change: stages of change and addictive behaviors. In: Miller W R, Heather N (eds) Treating addictive behaviours, 2nd edn. Plenum, New York

Heather N, Robertson I 1989 Problem drinking, 2nd edn. Oxford University Press, Oxford

Heather N, Rollnick S, Bell A, Richmond R 1996 Effects of brief counselling among male heavy drinkers identified on general hospital wards. Drug and Alcohol Review 15:29–38

Iveson G, Ratner H 1990 Problem to solution. Brief Therapy Press, London

Keller V, White M 1997 Choices and changes: a new model for influencing patient health behavior. Journal of Clinical Outcomes Management 4:33–36

Kemp R, Hayward P, Applewhaite G, Everitt B, David A 1996 Compliance therapy in psychotic patients: randomised controlled trial. British Medical Journal 312:345–349

Kuchipudi V, Hobein K, Flickinger A, Iber F L 1988 Failure of a 2-hour motivational intervention to alter recurrent drinking behaviour in alcoholics with gastrointestinal disease. Journal of Studies on Alcohol 51:356–360

Mann R E, Rollnick S 1996 Motivational interviewing with a sex offender who believed he was innocent. Behavioural and Cognitive Psychotherapy 24:127–134

Miller W R, Heather N (eds) 1998 Treating addictive behaviours, 2nd edn. Plenum, New York

Miller W R, Rollnick S 1991 Motivational interviewing: preparing people to change addictive behavior. Guilford Press, New York

Miller W, Sovereign G, Krege B 1988 Motivational interviewing with problem drinkers: II. The drinker's check-up as a preventative intervention. Behavioural Psychotherapy 16:251–268

Miller W, Benfield R, Tonigan S 1993 Enhancing motivation for change in problem drinking: a controlled comparison of two therapist styles. Journal of Consulting and Clinical Psychology 61:455–461

Ogden J 1996 Health psychology: a textbook. Open University Press: Buckingham

Pill R, Rees M (in press) Can nurses learn to let go? Issues arising from an intervention designed to improve patients' involvement in their own care. Journal of Advanced Nursing

Pill R, Stott N, Rollnick S, Rees M 1998 A randomised controlled trial of an intervention designed to improve the care given in general practice to type II diabetic patients: patient outcomes and professional ability to change behavior. Family Practice 15:229–235

Pinsof W M 1994 An overview of integrative problem centred therapy; a synthesis of family and individual psychotherapies. Journal of Family Therapy 16:103–120

Prochaska J O 1994 Strong and weak principles for progressing from precontemplation to action on the basis of twelve problem behaviours. Health Psychology 13:47–51

Prochaska J, DiClemente C 1983 Stages and processes of self-change of smoking: towards an integrated model of change. Journal of Consulting and Clinical Psychology 51:390–395

Prochaska J O, Velicer W F, Rossi J S et al 1994 Stages of change and decisional balance for 12 problem behaviors. Health Psychology 13:39–46

Prochaska J, DiClemente C 1998 Comments, criteria and creating better models: in response to Davidson. In: Miller W R, Heather N (eds) Treating addictive behaviours, 2nd edn. Plenum, New York

Project MATCH Research Group 1997 Matching Alcohol Treatment to Client Heterogenity: Project MATCH posttreatment drinking outcomes. Journal of Studies on Alcohol 58:7–29

Rollnick S 1998 Readiness, importance and confidence: critical conditions of change in treatment. In: Miller W R, Heather N (ed) Treating addictive behavior, 2nd edn. Plenum, New York

Rollnick S, Bell A 1991 Brief motivational interviewing for use by the non-specialist. In: Miller W R, Rollnick S (eds) Motivational interviewing: preparing people to change addictive behaviour. Guilford Press, New York

Rollnick S, Miller W R 1995 What is motivational interviewing? Behavioural and Cognitive Psychotherapy 23:325–334

Rollnick S, Heather N, Bell A 1992 Negotiating behaviour change in medical settings: the development of brief motivational interviewing. Journal of Mental Health 1:25–37

Rollnick S, Butler C C, Stott N 1997a Helping smokers make decisions: the enhancement of brief intervention for general medical practice. Patient Education and Counseling 31:191–203

Rollnick S, Butler C, Hodgson R 1997b Brief alcohol intervention in medical settings: concerns from the consulting room. Addiction Research 5:331–342

Russell M A H, Wilson C, Taylor C, Baker C D 1979 Effect of general practitioners' advice against smoking. British Medical Journal 2:231–235

Saunders W, Wilkinson C, Phillips M 1995 The impact of a brief motivational intervention with opiate users attending a methadone programme. Addiction 90:415–422

Schwarzer R, Fuchs R 1995 Changing risk behaviors and adopting health behaviors: the role of self-efficacy beliefs. In: Bandura A (ed) Self-efficacy in changing societies. Cambridge University Press, New York

Schwarzer R, Fuchs R 1996 Self-efficacy and health behaviours. In: Conner M, Norman P (eds) Predicting health behaviour: research and practice with social cognition models. Open University Press, Buckingham

Schmidt U, Treasure J 1997 Getting better bit(e) by bit(e): a survival kit for sufferers of bulimia nervosa and binge eating disorders. Clinician's Guide. Psychology Press, Hove

Senft R A, Polen M R, Freeborn D K, Hollis J F 1995 Drinking patterns and health. A randomized trial of screening and brief intervention in a primary care setting. Final report to the National Institute on Alcohol Abuse and Alcoholism, grant no. RO1-AA08976

Sesney J W, Kreher N E, Hickner J M, Webb S 1997 Smoking cessation interventions in rural family practices: an UPRNet study. Journal of Family Practice 44:578–585

Street E, Downey J 1996 Brief therapeutic consultations: an approach to systemic counselling. Wiley, Chichester

Stott N C H, Rollnick S, Rees M, Pill R 1995 Innovation in clinical method: diabetes care and negotiating skills. Family Practice 12:413–418

Stott N C H, Rees M, Rollnick S, Pill R, Hackett P 1996 Professional responses to innovation in clinical method: diabetes care and negotiation skills. Patient Education and Counseling 29:67–73

Stott N C H, Pill R M 1990 Advise yes, dictate no. Patients' views on health promotion in the consultation. Family Practice 7:125–131

Velicer W F, DiClemente C C, Prochaska J O, Brandenburg N 1985 Decisional balance measure for assessing and predicting smoking status. Journal of Personality and Social Psychology 48:1279–1289

Wallace P, Cutler S, Haines A 1988 Randomised controlled trial of general practitioner intervention in patients with excessive alcohol consumption. British Medical Journal 297:663–668

Wechsler H, Levine S, Idelson R K, Rohman M, Taylor J O 1983 The physician's role in health promotion: a survey of primary care physicians. New England Journal of Medicine 308:97–100

Index

Page numbers in bold refer to illustrations and tables